P9-CLX-868
3 1668 06950 9815

THE
EVERYTHING.
BIG BOOK OF FAT BOMBS

Dear Reader,

Two years ago I had a very rude awakening. It was the first time I measured my glucose levels, and I found out I was prediabetic.

At the age of forty-five I had been a nutritionist for five years and was eating what I thought was the healthiest diet on the planet: all organic, local, home-cooked, and Paleo foods. But something was not right . . . I was gaining weight. I was always hungry. I had joint and lower-back pain. Something had to change.

That is when I discovered the ketogenic diet. When designing my first ketogenic diet course for my patients, I started to feel the benefits of eating this way and completely fell in love with the keto lifestyle. Not only was I able to lose about fifteen pounds in three months (and I kept the weight off for the last three years!), I also since then reverted my prediabetes to normal blood sugar levels and I reset my insulin resistance so I can tolerate more carbs.

But that is not my favorite part of the diet. The variety and quality of the food you get to eat on a ketogenic lifestyle is my favorite part. No other way of eating promotes bacon, butter, and coconut oil. We all know that fat gives food its flavor, and since the keto diet focuses on consuming lots of fats, you know you'll be enjoying lots of great flavor too.

Fat bombs are a strategic invention to help you succeed with your keto lifestyle. They are an easy way to introduce more healthy fats into your day, which can be a daunting task, especially if you have been eating a low-fat diet for a long time!

In this book I have tried to bring the humble fat bomb up to the status of culinary genre so that you can benefit from a variety of flavors and ingredients, and stay motivated with keto!

Vivica Menegaz, CTWFN

Welcome to the EVERYTHING® Series!

These handy, accessible books give you all you need to tackle a difficult project, gain a new hobby, comprehend a fascinating topic, prepare for an exam, or even brush up on something you learned back in school but have since forgotten.

You can choose to read an Everything® book from cover to cover or just pick out the information you want from our four useful boxes: e-questions, e-facts, e-alerts, and e-ssentials. We give you everything you need to know on the subject, but throw in a lot of fun stuff along the way, too.

We now have more than 400 Everything® books in print, spanning such wide-ranging categories as weddings, pregnancy, cooking, music instruction, foreign language, crafts, pets, New Age, and so much more. When you're done reading them all, you can finally say you know Everything®!

PUBLISHER Karen Cooper

MANAGING EDITOR, EVERYTHING® SERIES Lisa Laing

COPY CHIEF Casey Ebert

ASSISTANT PRODUCTION EDITOR Jo-Anne Duhamel

ACQUISITIONS AND DEVELOPMENT EDITOR Hillary Thompson

EVERYTHING® SERIES COVER DESIGNER Erin Alexander

Visit the entire Everything® series at *www.everything.com*

THE
EVERYTHING®
Big Book of Fat Bombs

200

Irresistible Low-Carb, High-Fat Recipes
for Weight Loss the Ketogenic Way

Vivica Menegaz, CTWFN

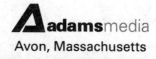

Avon, Massachusetts

I would like to dedicate this book to all the people who supported me in my journey to become a nutritionist. My parents, and my first mentor, Deborah Penner. Also my deep gratitude goes to my assistant Patty Woods, who made it possible for this book to become a reality.

Copyright © 2016 by F+W Media, Inc.
All rights reserved.
This book, or parts thereof, may not be reproduced in any form without permission from the publisher; exceptions are made for brief excerpts used in published reviews.

An Everything® Series Book.
Everything® and everything.com® are registered trademarks of F+W Media, Inc.

Published by
Adams Media, a division of F+W Media, Inc.
57 Littlefield Street, Avon, MA 02322. U.S.A.
www.adamsmedia.com

Contains material adapted from *The Everything® Guide to the Ketogenic Diet* by Lindsay Boyers, copyright © 2015 by F+W Media, Inc., ISBN 10: 1-4405-8691-8, ISBN 13: 978-1-4405-8691-0.

ISBN 10: 1-4405-9675-1
ISBN 13: 978-1-4405-9675-9
eISBN 10: 1-4405-9676-X
eISBN 13: 978-1-4405-9676-6

Printed in the United States of America.

10 9 8 7 6 5 4 3 2 1

The information in this book should not be used for diagnosing or treating any health problem. Not all diet and exercise plans suit everyone. You should always consult a trained medical professional before starting a diet, taking any form of medication, or embarking on any fitness or weight-training program. The author and publisher disclaim any liability arising directly or indirectly from the use of this book.

Always follow safety and commonsense cooking protocol while using kitchen utensils, operating ovens and stoves, and handling uncooked food. If children are assisting in the preparation of any recipe, they should always be supervised by an adult.

Many of the designations used by manufacturers and sellers to distinguish their products are claimed as trademarks. Where those designations appear in this book and F+W Media, Inc. was aware of a trademark claim, the designations have been printed with initial capital letters.

Cover photos by Vivica Menegaz.
Nutritional statistics by Nicole Cormier, RD, LDN.

This book is available at quantity discounts for bulk purchases.
For information, please call 1-800-289-0963.

Contents

Introduction

The ketogenic diet, despite being around for decades, has gained plenty of popularity recently. This is no surprise, considering the benefits of this diet reach far beyond its original medical goal of seizure control. Created in the 1920s to control epileptic seizures in young children, this diet helped children manage symptoms and cope with seizures. Once antiseizure drugs were invented, however, the diet fell off the medical map. Body builders later rediscovered the ketogenic diet and began using it to achieve remarkably lean body composition before competitions.

One of the main benefits of burning ketones for energy is that they are a highly stable and long-lasting energy source, like a smooth freeway, unlike the crazy energy rollercoaster ride of a glucose-fueled diet. When eating a ketogenic diet, blood sugars gradually stabilize, so hunger quickly subsides, mood brightens, and energy improves.

The almost complete absence of hunger pangs makes this way of eating ideal if you're looking to lose weight. Using fat as the primary fuel source enables the body to easily access stored fat reserves and use them for fuel with great efficiency. Those who follow a true ketogenic diet often lose weight rapidly because of this.

Fat burning increases and stabilizes energy. The brain loves ketones; they are like high-octane gasoline for brain functions, eliminating "brain fog" and sharpening cognitive functions. That is why this diet works as an ideal prevention for cognitive dysfunctions like Alzheimer's disease. Another major benefit of this diet is the reduction of inflammation in the body, resulting in a substantial reduction of pain and other unpleasant symptoms.

Starting a keto lifestyle might seem challenging, especially when you're not used to eating fat. It doesn't help that doctors and the media have told people for years that fat is the enemy, while in truth, the real enemy is the consumption of high levels of sugar and carbs. Once people have a mindset shift back to the appreciation of healthy fats, they will realize that this diet is really based on flavor and pleasure, not deprivation and sacrifice, like most low-fat diets.

Fat bombs definitively belong in the category of fun, pleasurable foods. Fat bombs were created as a high-fat, no-carbohydrate snack designed to increase the amount of good fats in a keto diet. In this book, the humble fat bomb is elevated to its own culinary genre, transcending the definition of a snack and becoming a meal itself.

Savory fat bombs are the best ally to keep pesky sugar cravings under control, and sweet fat bombs will indulge the senses and anchor blood sugars to a steady low number! Some of the fat bombs are really a small meal in themselves, designed to accommodate the demands of busy lifestyles. They can be made ahead of time and are easily stored in the refrigerator for few days.

Sweet fat bombs double as great desserts for family and friends, or good healthy snacks for kids. And many of the recipes in this book are dairy-free to accommodate Keto Paleo and Paleo readers. Avoiding dairy is important when you have food sensitivities, so your body can start the process of healing. Now everyone can enjoy the benefits of this way of eating and stay away from highly processed and sugary foods.

Using fat bombs will enable you to stay true to a ketogenic way of life. The fat bomb is truly the secret weapon every healthy eater should have in his or her arsenal to eat clean, stay full, and feel absolutely satisfied instead of deprived.

Acknowledgments

I would like to acknowledge Hillary Thompson for her support and guidance with the production of the book. I would also like to say thank you to all my patients and readers, whose constant feedback helped create better and better recipes for healing.

CHAPTER 1

Understanding Ketosis

Your body is highly intelligent. It knows exactly what it wants, and knows exactly what it needs to do to get what it wants. What your body wants is energy. Without energy, your cells starve and you die. Your body has several metabolic pathways it can use to convert the food you eat into energy. The default metabolic pathway uses glucose from carbohydrates consumed as fuel. As long as you provide your body with carbohydrates, it uses them as energy while storing the excess as fat in the process. When you deny your body carbohydrates, it needs to get the energy somewhere else to survive.

What Is Ketosis?

Your body's second preferred source of energy is fat. When carbohydrates are not easily accessible, your body turns to fat to get vital energy. The liver will break down fat into fatty acids, which then break down into an energy-rich substance called ketones. When your body burns fats instead of carbohydrates for energy, the process is called ketosis. The goal of a ketogenic diet is to kick your body into long-term ketosis, ultimately turning it into a fat-burning machine.

How Your Body Obtains Energy

Your cells need a constant supply of energy. Even when you're sitting on the couch, your body is generating energy for your cells. Since energy cannot be created, only converted from one form to another, your body gets this energy from the food you eat or from its own energy reserves, your body fat. Your body can use each macronutrient (carbohydrates, fat, and protein) for energy. The bio-chemical process of obtaining energy is a complicated one, but it's important to understand a few basics to get a feel for how ketosis works on a cellular level.

Energy from Protein

Protein is the body's least favorite macronutrient to use as energy since it serves so many other functions in the body. Protein provides structural support to every cell in your body and helps maintain your body tissues. Proteins also act as enzymes that play a role in all of the chemical reactions in your body. Without these enzymes, these chemical reactions would be so slow that your body wouldn't be able to carry out basic processes like digestion and metabolism that are necessary for survival. Proteins also help maintain fluid and acid-base balance, help transport substances such as oxygen through the body and waste out of the body, and act as antibodies to fight off illness.

 Essential

This process of using protein for energy is what makes extreme calorie restriction dangerous. When your diet doesn't provide enough calories, your body begins to break down the protein in your muscles for energy, which can lead to muscle loss or muscle wasting in addition to nutritional deficiencies.

Proteins are made up of amino acids. When you eat proteins, your body breaks them down into their individual amino acids, which are then converted into sugars through a process called deamination. Your body can use these protein-turned-sugars as a form of energy, but that means your body isn't using the amino acids for those other important functions. It's best to avoid forcing the body to use protein for energy, and you do that by providing it with the other nutrients it needs. That being said, if the body has no other choice but to use protein for energy, it will.

Energy from Carbohydrates

Although your body is adept at using any food that's available for energy, it always turns to carbohydrates first. When you eat carbohydrates, they are broken down into glucose or another sugar that's easily converted to glucose. Glucose is absorbed through the walls of the small intestine and then enters your body by way of your bloodstream, which causes your blood glucose levels to rise. As soon as the glucose enters your blood, your pancreas sends out insulin to pick up the sugar and carry it to your cells so they can use it as energy.

Once your cells have used all the glucose they need at that time, much of the remaining glucose is converted into glycogen so it can be stored in the liver and muscles. The liver has a limited ability to store glycogen, though. It can only store enough glycogen to provide you with energy for about twenty-four hours. All the extra glucose that can't be stored or burned is converted into triglycerides, which are stored in your fat cells.

 Fact

A healthy adult can store about 500 grams (2,000 calories worth) of carbohydrates. Approximately 400 grams are stored as glycogen in your muscles, 90–110 grams are stored as glycogen in the liver, and 25 grams circulate throughout the bloodstream as glucose. However, your body has an unlimited ability to store fat.

When you don't eat for a few hours and your blood sugar starts to drop, your body will call on the glycogen stored in the liver and muscles for energy before anything else. The pancreas releases a hormone called glucagon that triggers the release of glucose from the glycogen stored in your liver to help raise your blood sugar levels. This process is called glycogenolysis. The glycogen stored in your liver is used exclusively to increase your blood glucose levels, while the glycogen stored in your muscles is used strictly as fuel for your muscles. When you eat carbohydrates again, your body uses the glucose it gets from them to replenish those glycogen stores. If you regularly eat carbohydrates, your body never has a problem getting access to glucose for energy, and the stored fat stays where it is—in your fat cells.

 Fact

Endurance athletes use the terms "hitting a wall" or "bonking" to describe the point at which they've depleted their glycogen stores and no longer have access to a quick form of energy. Bonking usually manifests as sudden fatigue or a complete loss of energy. When you see marathon runners drinking glucose shots during a race, it's because they want to replenish glycogen stores quickly so that they have enough energy to finish.

Energy from Fat

The body prefers to use carbohydrates for energy because they're easily accessible and fast acting, but in the absence of carbohydrates, your body turns to fat. The fat from the food you eat is broken down into fatty acids, which enter the bloodstream through the walls of the small intestine. Most of your cells can directly use fatty acids for energy, but some specialized cells, such as the cells in your brain and your muscles, can't run on fatty acids directly. To appease these cells and give them the energy they need, your body uses fatty acids to make ketones.

The Creation of Ketones

When your body doesn't have access to glucose, (i.e., during times of fasting or when intentionally following a low-carbohydrate diet) it turns to fat for energy. Fat is taken to the liver where it is broken down into glycerol and fatty acids through a process called beta-oxidation. The fatty-acid molecules are further broken down through a process called ketogenesis, and a specific ketone body called acetoacetate is formed.

Over time, as your body becomes adapted to using ketones as fuel, your muscles convert acetoacetate into beta-hydroxybutyrate, or BHB, which is the preferred ketogenic source of energy for your brain, and acetone, most of which is expelled from the body as waste.

The glycerol created during beta-oxidation goes through a process called gluconeogenesis. During gluconeogenesis, the body converts glycerol into glucose that your body can use for energy. Your body can also convert excess protein into glucose. Your body does need some glucose to function, but it doesn't need carbohydrates to get it. It does a good job of converting whatever it can into the simple sugar.

Ketosis and Weight Loss

Now that you understand how your body creates energy and how ketones are formed, you may be left wondering how this translates into weight loss. When you eat a lot of carbohydrates, your body happily burns them for energy and stores any excess as glycogen in your liver or as triglycerides in your fat cells. When you take carbohydrates out of the equation, your body depletes its glycogen stores in the liver and muscles and then turns to fat for energy. Your body obtains energy from the fat in the food you eat, but it also uses the triglycerides, or fats, stored in your fat cells.

 Essential

Triglycerides are the storage form of fat in your body from the food you eat. When you eat more food than your body needs for energy, it is converted into triglycerides and stored in your fat cells for later use.

When your body starts burning stored fat, your fat cells shrink and you begin to lose weight and become leaner. Of course, in order for that to happen, you will have to reduce your caloric intake, as your body will otherwise store the fat you eat as well.

How to Induce Ketosis

Inducing ketosis is not always an easy task, but once you get the hang of it, it can become second nature. The first step in inducing ketosis is to severely limit carbohydrate consumption, but that's not quite enough. You must limit your protein consumption as well. Traditional low-carbohydrate diets don't induce ketosis because they allow a high intake of protein. Because your body is able to convert excess protein into glucose, your body never switches over to burning fat as fuel. You can induce ketosis by following a ketogenic diet—one that is high in fat and allows moderate amounts of protein with a small amount of carbohydrates.

The exact percentage of each macronutrient you need to force your body into ketosis may vary from person to person, but in general, the macronutrient ratio falls into the following ranges:

- 60–75 percent of calories from fat
- 15–30 percent of calories from protein
- 5–10 percent of calories from carbohydrates

This largely differs from the standard low-carbohydrate diet, which typically allows more calories to come from protein, and the traditional dietary reference intakes set by the Institute of Medicine.

Currently, the Institute of Medicine recommends getting 45–65 percent of your calories from carbohydrates, 20–35 percent of your calories from fat, and 10–35 percent of your calories from protein. Although the individual recommendations of low-carbohydrate diets differ based on which one you follow, they typically allow about 20 percent of calories from carbohydrates, 25–30 percent from protein, and 55–65 percent from fat.

Once you're in ketosis, you have to continue with the high-fat, low-carbohydrate, moderate-protein plan. Eating too many carbohydrates or too much protein can kick you out of ketosis at any time by providing your body with enough glucose to stop using fat as fuel.

Signs That You Are in Ketosis

Signs that you're in ketosis may start appearing after only one week of following a true ketogenic diet. For some people, it can take longer—as much as three weeks. The amount of time it takes for you to start seeing signs that your body is burning fat for fuel largely depends on you as an individual. When signs do start to show, they are pretty similar across the board.

Keto "Flu"

"Keto flu" or "low-carb flu" commonly affects people in the first few days of starting a ketogenic diet. Of course, the ketogenic diet doesn't actually cause the flu, but the phenomenon is given the term because its symptoms closely resemble that of the flu. It would be more accurate to refer to this stage as a carbohydrate withdrawal, because that's really what it is. When you take carbohydrates away, it causes altered hormonal states and electrolyte imbalances that are responsible for the associated symptoms. The basic symptoms include headache, nausea, upset stomach, sleepiness, fatigue, abdominal cramps, diarrhea, and lack of mental clarity, or what is commonly referred to as "brain fog."

 Fact

Carbohydrate addiction is a real thing. Some research shows that carbohydrates activate certain stimuli in the brain that can be dependence forming. Carbohydrate addicts have uncontrollable cravings, and when they do eat, they tend to binge. In a carbohydrate addict, the removal of carbohydrates can cause withdrawal symptoms, such as dizziness and irritability, and intense cravings.

The duration of symptoms varies—it depends on you as an individual—but typically a "keto flu" lasts anywhere from a couple of days to a week. In rare cases, it can last up to two weeks. Some of the symptoms of the "keto flu" are associated with dehydration, because in the beginning stages of ketosis you lose a lot of water weight. With that lost fluid, you also lose electrolytes. You can replenish these electrolytes by drinking enhanced waters (but make sure they are not sweetened) and drinking lots of homemade bone broth. This may help lessen the severity of the symptoms.

Bad Breath

Unfortunately, bad breath is another early sign that you're in ketosis. When you're in ketosis, your body creates acetone as a waste product. Some of this acetone is released in your breath, giving it a fruity or ammonia-like quality. You can combat bad breath by chewing on fresh mint leaves and drinking plenty of water, since bad breath is also associated with dehydration.

Decreased Appetite and Nausea

As your body adapts to a ketogenic diet, you may have a decreased appetite. This is because you're providing your body with plenty of fat and protein, which are both highly satiating, and not a lot of carbohydrates. The nausea associated with "keto adapting" can also decrease your appetite. When you reach this stage, it's important that you eat regularly, even if you feel like you aren't hungry. You want to make sure your body is getting enough nutrients and maintaining steady blood sugar levels, especially in this time of transition.

Increased Energy

When the fog begins to clear and your body starts to become keto-adapted, the uncomfortable symptoms you felt will dissipate and you'll start seeing the benefits of following a ketogenic diet. One of the first beneficial signs many people experience is an increase in energy. When your body breaks down fat instead of carbohydrates, more energy is produced gram for gram, leaving you feeling alert and energized. Also stable blood sugar levels avoid the rushes and crashes of excess carbohydrate consumption, giving you a stable, enduring source of energy.

Improved Focus and Mental Clarity

Many mental issues, such as brain fog and problems with memory, are caused by what is called neurotoxicity, the exposure of the nervous system to toxic substances. For the brain, exposure to too much glucose can result in neurotoxicity. When you reduce the supply of glucose in your body and your brain starts to use ketones as fuel, the toxicity levels diminish. As a result, you may be able to think more clearly, focus better, and have better memory recall.

Other Possible Signs

Other possible signs of ketosis include:

- Cold hands and feet
- Increased urinary frequency
- Difficulty sleeping
- Metallic taste in the mouth
- Dry mouth
- Increased thirst

Measurable Ketones

Your body is pretty good at letting you know when you're in ketosis without any testing, but if you want to be absolutely sure, you can test your ketone levels with urine strips or a blood meter. Urine strips allow you to easily test for the presence of ketones in your urine, while blood meters can test for ketones with a small blood sample from a prick in your finger. These testing methods tend to be more reliable than just trusting the presence of symptoms. If you really want to know if you're producing ketones, these tests are a great way to find out. Keep in mind that some methods are more reliable than others. For example, urine strips are a great way to test at the beginning of ketosis, but they become unreliable once you have keto-adapted.

Although these signs are common among many people who follow a ketogenic diet, your experience may be different. Everybody is unique, so it's impossible to say exactly what your personal experience will be. Keep in mind that in the early stages of ketosis your symptoms may be unpleasant, but as your body adapts you will begin to experience the benefits of following a ketogenic diet plan.

 Fact

During the first few weeks on the ketogenic diet your body undergoes a series of changes to adapt its functions for burning fat as the preferred fuel source. This process is called *keto adaptation*. Some of these adaptations include adapting the brain to burn ketones instead of glucose. The brain will be able to use a maximum of 75 percent ketones for energy; the rest will always have to be glucose. As stated, the body will be able to produce its own glucose from protein and triglycerides.

Managing Uncomfortable Symptoms

The initial symptoms of a ketogenic diet are uncomfortable, but if you choose to ride it out, rest assured, in time, they will go away. If the thought of being uncomfortable is really too much to bear, there are a few things you can try to help decrease the chances of experiencing symptoms, or at least lessen their severity.

Start Slowly

Like anything else, symptoms tend to be the worst when you transition to a ketogenic diet cold turkey. If you've been following a high-carbohydrate, low-fat diet for years—even decades—abruptly asking your body to run on fat instead is like a slap in the face. Instead of jumping right into a ketogenic diet, transition slowly.

Start by gradually eliminating non-nutritive carbohydrate sources, such as soda, desserts, sugary snacks, pasta, and pizza, over a period of a few weeks. As you eliminate these carbohydrate sources, increase the amount of fats you eat—coconut, avocado, and cheese, for example. When you've gotten used to the general principles of the diet, start tracking specific numbers and macronutrient ratios.

Snack Regularly

Eating a high-fat or a fat-protein snack, such as a fat bomb, will help stabilize your blood sugars during the initial phases of keto adaptation, so it will help ease certain symptoms, including headache and irritability. When you're first starting a ketogenic diet, make sure to snack regularly to keep yourself from getting too hungry.

Drink Water

Many of the symptoms, such as bad breath, are associated with being dehydrated. Drink plenty of water while you're transitioning and for the entire duration of your ketogenic diet. To make sure you stay hydrated, add a pinch of Celtic sea salt or Himalayan salt to every glass of water you drink. It won't taste salty, but it provides you with essential electrolytes.

Drink Bone Broth

Drinking homemade bone broth will also provide needed electrolytes to the body. It can be beef, chicken, lamb, or even fish broth. Drink about 3–4 cups a day for best results.

CHAPTER 2

The Ketogenic Diet

Now that you have a full understanding of how the body obtains energy and what ketosis is (a state during which your body relies on fat for energy instead of carbohydrates), it's time to put all that information to good use. As the name implies, the ketogenic diet is a diet plan that puts your body's innate intelligence to work by forcing your body to enter into a state of ketosis. Your body already instinctively knows how to do this when you don't eat carbohydrates, but the point of the ketogenic diet is to force it to happen and keep it going for as long as you want. If you're interested in starting a ketogenic diet, a qualified nutrition or healthcare professional can help you get started.

What Is the Ketogenic Diet?

The ketogenic diet encourages you to get most of your calories from fat and severely restrict carbohydrates. Unlike a typical low-carbohydrate diet, the ketogenic diet is not a high-protein diet. Instead, it's a high-fat, moderate-protein, and low-carbohydrate diet. Although your exact macronutrient ratio will differ based on your individual needs, a typical nutritional ketogenic diet looks something like this:

- Fat: 60–75 percent of calories
- Protein: 15–30 percent of calories
- Carbohydrates: 5–10 percent of calories

These are just general guidelines, but most people on a successful ketogenic diet fall somewhere in this range. In order to figure what you should be eating, you'll have to calculate your individual macronutrient ratios. As your diet progresses and your body begins to change, you may have to recalculate these numbers and make the proper adjustments to your diet plan.

Calculating Your Macronutrient Ratio

The first thing you need to do to calculate your macronutrient ratio is figure out how many calories you should be eating. There are several online calculators that can calculate this number for you, but to do it yourself, you can use a method called the Mifflin-St. Jeor formula, which looks like this:

- *Men:*
  $10 \times$ weight (kg) $+ 6.25 \times$ height (cm) $- 5 \times$ age (y) $+ 5$
- *Women:*
  $10 \times$ weight (kg) $+ 6.25 \times$ height (cm) $- 5 \times$ age (y) $- 161$

To make this explanation easier, let's try using the equation with a thirty-year-old, 160-pound (72.7 kg) woman who is 5 feet 5 inches (165.1 cm) tall. When you plug this woman's statistics into the Mifflin-St. Jeor formula, you can see that she should be eating 1,448 calories per day. Now you'll use the estimated macronutrient percentages to calculate how much of each nutrient she needs to consume in order to follow a successful ketogenic diet plan.

Carbohydrates

On a ketogenic diet, carbohydrates should provide only 5–10 percent of the calories you consume. Many ketogenic dieters stay at the low end of 5 percent, but the exact amount you need depends on your body. Unfortunately, there is no one-size-fits-all approach to this, so you'll have to do a little trial and error. You can pick a percentage that feels right for you and try that out for a couple of weeks. If you don't see the results you want, you'll have to adjust your nutrient ratios and calculate them again. Getting 7 percent of your calories from carbohydrates is a good place to start.

To calculate how many grams of carbohydrates this is, multiply 7 percent by the total number of calories, which, in the earlier example, is 1,448 and then divide by 4 (since carbohydrates contain 4 calories per gram). The number you're left with is the amount of carbohydrates in grams you should eat per day. In this example, the number is 25 grams.

Total Carbohydrates versus Net Carbohydrates

When counting carbohydrates on a ketogenic diet plan, you want to pay attention to net carbohydrates, not total carbohydrates. Net carbohydrates are the amount of carbohydrates left over after you subtract grams of fiber from total grams of carbohydrates. If a particular food contains 10 grams of carbohydrates, but 7 grams come from fiber, the total number of net carbohydrates is 3 grams. You count the 3 grams toward your daily total rather than the 10 grams.

This is a general rule that works for most people. In the case of diabetes or high insulin resistance you might have to start by counting whole carbs instead, as you might be sensitive to the fiber part of the carbohydrate.

Fat

After you've calculated carbohydrates, move on to fat. Again, the exact amount you'll need depends on you as an individual, but consuming 75 percent of your calories from fat is a good place to start. To figure out the amount of fat you need in grams, multiply the amount of calories you need (in this example, 1,448) by 75 percent and then divide by 9 (since fat contains 9 calories per gram). The number you're left with is the total grams of fat you need for the day. In this example, it's 121 grams.

Remember that fat is what fills the caloric need on a ketogenic diet, so if your goal is to lose weight, you will be reducing the amount of fat you eat.

Protein

Once you've calculated carbohydrates and fat, protein is easy. The remainder of your calories, which equates to 18 percent, should come from protein. To figure out this number in grams, multiply the total number of calories by 18 percent and then divide by 4 (since protein contains 4 calories per gram). The number you're left with is the total grams of protein you need for the day. In this example, it's 65 grams.

 Essential

As your body changes, your macronutrient ranges may also change. When following a ketogenic diet, it's beneficial to recalculate your nutrient needs regularly—about once per month. If your needs change, adjust your diet accordingly.

Foods to Eat and Avoid

When following a ketogenic diet, some foods are strictly off-limits, while others fall into a sort of gray area. Regardless of whether foods are "allowed," you still have to make sure that you're staying within your macronutrient ratios. Just because a food is technically allowed doesn't mean you can eat as much of it as you want. Use these recommendations as a guideline, but always make sure that you're staying within your calculated macronutrient ratios.

The Meaning of Keto Paleo

You can basically eat a ketogenic diet and eat fast food every day. Ketogenic, after all, only means a certain ratio of macronutrients designed to induce ketosis. That would not be eating for your health, though.

If you want to maximize the benefits of eating a ketogenic diet, you should also choose whole, unprocessed, fresh foods as much as possible. Keto Paleo means eliminating all highly processed foods, artificial sweeteners, and dairy. Keto Primal includes dairy, which is a valid option if you do not have any food sensitivity or have no trouble losing weight.

Choosing the Best Ingredients

The quality of your food matters, especially when it comes to fat and protein sources. Ideally, you want to choose meats that are organic, grassfed, and pasture raised. Eggs should come from your local farmer or from pasture-raised hens whenever possible. Choose grassfed butter and organic creams, cheese, fruits, and vegetables. Eating conventional foods won't prevent you from entering a ketogenic state, but high-quality foods are better for your body in general. After all, you are what you eat. Do your best to get the highest-quality food you can find and/or afford.

Fats and Oils

Fats and oils provide the basis of your ketogenic diet, so you'll want to make sure you're eating plenty of them. The ketogenic diet is not just a fat free-for-all, though. While following a ketogenic diet, there are certain fats that are better for you than others, although which ones fall into which category may surprise you. On the ketogenic diet, you should eat plenty of saturated fats in the form of meat, poultry, eggs, butter, and coconut; monounsaturated fats, such as olive oil, nuts, nut butters, and avocado; and natural polyunsaturated fats, such as tuna, salmon, and mackerel. Avoid highly processed polyunsaturated fats, such as canola oil, vegetable oil, and soybean oil. Homemade mayonnaise is also an easy way to add a dose of fat to every meal.

Proteins

Many of the fat sources mentioned previously—meat, poultry, eggs, butter, nuts, nut butters, and fish—are also loaded with protein and should be your main protein sources when following a ketogenic diet. Bacon and sausage are other sources of protein that also provide a significant dose of fat. When eating protein make sure to stay within your recommended grams for the day, since your body turns excess protein into glucose, which can kick you out of ketosis.

Fruits and Vegetables

When following a ketogenic diet, most fruits fall onto the "do not eat" list. Even though the sugars in fruit are natural sugars, they still raise your blood glucose levels significantly and can kick you out of ketosis. There's not a hard rule that fruit isn't allowed on a ketogenic diet, but you do need to limit your intake. When you do eat fruit, choose fruits that are high in fiber and lower in carbohydrates, such as berries, and limit your portions.

Vegetables are extremely important on a ketogenic diet. They provide the vitamins and minerals that you need to stay healthy and help fill you up without contributing a lot of calories to your day. You do have to be choosy about which vegetables you eat, though, since some are loaded with carbohydrates and do not have a place on a ketogenic diet. As a general rule, choose dark green or leafy green vegetables, such as spinach, broccoli, cucumbers, green beans, lettuce, and asparagus. Cauliflower and mushrooms are also good choices for a ketogenic diet. Avoid starchy vegetables, including white potatoes, sweet potatoes, yams, and corn.

Dairy

Dairy products can be an easy way to add fat to your diet. If you have no history of food sensitivities and have no known insulin resistance, dairy can be a good option for you. Full-fat, organic dairy products are very suited to a ketogenic diet. Use butter, heavy cream, sour cream, cream cheese, hard cheese, and cottage cheese to help meet your fat needs. Avoid low-fat dairy products and flavored dairy products, such as fruity yogurt. Flavored yogurt is full of sugar; serving for serving, some versions contain as much sugar and carbohydrates as soda.

Beverages

As with any diet plan, when it comes to beverages, water is your best bet. Make sure to drink at least half of your body weight in ounces. Coffee and tea are also permitted on a ketogenic diet, but they must be unsweetened or sweetened with an approved sweetener, such as stevia or erythritol. Avoid sodas, flavored waters, sweetened teas, sweetened lemonade, and fruit juices. You can infuse plain water with fresh herbs, such as mint or basil, to give yourself a little variety.

Grains and Sugars

Avoid grains and sugars in all of their forms on the ketogenic diet. Grains include wheat, barley, rice, rye, sorghum, and anything made from these products. That means no breads, no pasta, no crackers, and no rice. Sugar, and anything that contains sugar, is also not allowed on a ketogenic diet. This includes white sugar, brown sugar, honey, maple syrup, corn syrup, and brown rice syrup. There are many names for sugar on ingredient lists; it's extremely beneficial to familiarize yourself with these names so you'll know when a product contains sugar in any form.

Starting a Ketogenic Diet

If you're used to following a standard American diet—one in which most of your calories come from carbohydrates—a ketogenic diet is a major change. You have two choices: jump into it cold turkey, or slowly wean yourself off carbohydrates by increasing your fat intake until your macronutrient ratios fall within your goal. When you go into it cold turkey, you're more likely to experience unpleasant carbohydrate withdrawal symptoms, so easing into it slowly is often the best bet for success.

Carbohydrate Guides

Carbohydrate guides are a helpful tool to use with the ketogenic diet, especially when you're just starting out. Many books are available that provide a list of foods and their carbohydrate count (as well as their calorie, protein, and fat content). Some of these books categorize foods into high-carbohydrate, medium-carbohydrate, and low-carbohydrate lists. There are also several mobile apps that do the same thing.

Whatever method you choose, make sure you have your carbohydrate guide handy when you're food shopping so you can double-check what foods are allowed on the diet and which foods aren't. As you get the hang of the diet, you won't need to check every single food before you purchase it, but it's still handy to have the guides easily accessible for those once in a while foods that you're unsure about.

Prepare Your Kitchen

Once you've made the decision to start a ketogenic diet, you need to prepare your kitchen. This is a two-part process: You'll need to remove off-plan foods, and you need to stock your refrigerator and pantry with the essentials. If you live alone or with others who are also following a ketogenic diet, removing off-plan foods is simple. Go through your pantry and refrigerator and take out all the foods that don't fit into your diet plan. Don't forget to check the labels on your spices and dried herbs. Sometimes these contain sugar, gluten, or other artificial ingredients that don't belong on a ketogenic diet. Donate unopened items to your local food pantry and toss the open ones in the trash.

If you're the only one in your household starting a ketogenic diet, this removal process is a little more complicated. Instead of donating or throwing out foods that are off-plan, divide the pantry up. If possible, put all ketogenic-approved foods in a separate cabinet and make it a point to only go in there and not even look in the off-plan cabinet. Dividing up the refrigerator might be even more difficult than dividing the pantry, but do the best you can to separate what you can eat from what you can't.

The second part of preparing your kitchen is to stock up on all the essentials. It's imperative that you always have foods on hand that you can eat. If you don't, you're more likely to get to the point of being so hungry that you'll eat anything.

Ease Into It

When you're excited about starting a new diet, it's tempting to jump right in, but your body will thank you if you ease it into the ketogenic diet slowly. Doing so will lessen the severity of any of the "keto flu" symptoms you might experience and make the transition a little easier. Give yourself about three to four weeks from the time you commit to following a ketogenic diet to the day you actually start it 100 percent.

 Alert

Although artificially sweetened beverages are allowed on a ketogenic diet because they don't contain any carbohydrates, they are not Keto Paleo and they are definitively not good for you. Some research shows that even though artificial sweeteners don't contain any calories, they can contribute to weight gain. Plus, part of the goal is to try to get rid of your sweet tooth, and drinking sweetened beverages won't help you do that.

During the first week, cut out all sugary beverages. This includes soda, lemonade, sweetened teas, and flavored waters. If you put sugar in your coffee, scale back—use one teaspoon instead of two. After one week of this, remove all desserts and sugary snacks from your diet, including candy, cookies, cakes, muffins, chocolates, and ice cream. This might be a good time to start making some sweet fat bombs and using them as a substitute for sugary sweets, to ease your transition. Get in the habit of not having dessert after dinner. You want to train your body to stop craving sweets, so starting to substitute them for sugar-free sweets is an important first step. On your third week, cut out starchy carbohydrates such as pasta, pizza, bread, crackers, rolls, and potatoes. At this point, you may have already started to lose weight.

When you start week four, you'll be ready to officially start your ketogenic diet. This is when you should start tracking your macronutrients to make sure you're staying within the correct ratios. Limiting carbohydrates is important, but it's not the only goal; make sure you're also eating plenty of fat and moderate amounts of protein.

 Essential

Years ago, unless you had the fancy, expensive software that nutritionists use, the only way to track your macronutrients was by looking up each food item; writing down its carbohydrate, protein, and fat content; and adding it all up. Nowadays, there are several apps that you can download on your phone that will do the work for you. Make your life easier by downloading one of these apps—a popular one is MyFitnessPal—and tracking everything you eat.

Stay Hydrated and Replenish Electrolytes

Staying hydrated is always important, but it's especially vital when you're starting a ketogenic diet. It's not only about drinking water; you also want to replenish your electrolytes. When you start a ketogenic diet, you initially lose water, which takes electrolytes such as sodium and potassium with it. Aim to drink the equivalent of at least half your body weight in ounces. This means that, for example, if you're 180 pounds, you'll want to drink at least 90 ounces of water a day.

 Essential

The soup stocks and broths that you get at the store are a lot different from the bone broth you make at home. To make an electrolyte-rich bone broth, get some high-quality soup bones from your local farmer or butcher. Put these bones in a pot and add enough water to just cover them. Add some salt and pepper, and some bay leaves if you prefer, and let the broth simmer for 12–24 hours. You can also make broth with a whole chicken and some herbs and let that simmer 8–12 hours.

You can replenish your electrolytes by drinking a cup of home-made bone broth every day, by adding salt to your foods, and by adding a pinch of salt to your drinking water.

Planning Meals for Long-Term Success

Planning your meals is vital to your long-term success on a ketogenic diet. There is a popular quote, most often credited to Benjamin Franklin, that goes something like this: "When you fail to plan, you plan to fail." It's true. The best way to ensure success is to plan your weekly meals, prepare meals in advance, and always make sure you have ketogenic-approved snacks on hand, like the fat bombs contained in this guide.

Meal Planning

Take one night a week and write out everything you will eat all week. Plan your meals and your snacks and then compile a grocery list for what you'll need in order to execute these meals and snacks. You may choose to make your meal-planning day your shopping day as well. Get everything you need in one swoop and then don't stray from your plan.

Meal Prep

Once you know what you're going to eat all week, you may decide that you want to cook each meal individually, or you may decide that spending a few hours prepping your meals makes more sense for you. If you choose the latter, pick a day when you don't have any other commitments and spend a few hours in the kitchen preparing your meals for the entire week. You can make a quiche, a couple of ketogenic-friendly casseroles, and a big pot of soup. Divide each meal into to-go containers and store them in the refrigerator so that they're ready to go when you are.

Being Prepared

When you're on a specialized diet such as the ketogenic one, there is really no such thing as convenience foods. You have to be prepared at all times. You might have to take meals and snacks with you everywhere you go, but it's a small price to pay for the way you'll feel. Pack a lunch every day and keep nonperishable snacks like fat bombs, coconut shavings, nuts, and seeds in your car, in your desk at work, and in your purse or briefcase.

Don't Make It Complicated

It's tempting to want to create elaborate meal plans that feature a new gourmet entrée each night, but for most people that's just not realistic. You have to make sure that your new diet plan can fit into your lifestyle; otherwise, you won't be able to stick to it. Keep things simple by eating the same thing for breakfast three times a week and using leftovers from dinner for the next day's lunch. You can double or triple recipes to prepare meals in bulk and then freeze them for another day when you don't have the time to cook.

Starting a new diet is not easy; it takes dedication and preparation. You'll have to do some fine-tuning and rearranging to figure out what works for you, but once you get the hang of it, it will become second nature.

CHAPTER 3

Fat and the Fat Bomb

If you're one of the people who followed a low-fat diet and failed to lose weight, or failed to see any other major health improvements, don't worry; you're in the company of millions. When the popularity of the low-fat diet surged, many followers found themselves gaining more weight. Removing fat from your diet was supposed to make you thinner and healthier, but it did just the opposite. When people started replacing fats with carbohydrates and low-fat alternatives, the incidences of diabetes and obesity began to skyrocket. Could the beloved low-fat diet be to blame? Absolutely.

Low-Fat Diet Myths

If you're still on the low-fat diet train, read this next sentence carefully and really let it sink in: Fat is not your enemy; sugar is. And that applies to all forms of sugar, not only the granulated stuff that you put in your coffee in the morning. Sure, the sugar in fruit is packaged with vitamin C, potassium, fiber, and other valuable nutrients, which makes it a far superior choice over regular old sugar, but overdoing it can actually hinder weight-loss efforts and set you up for more serious conditions like diabetes and cardiovascular disease. But before delving too deeply into sugar, it's important to spend some time debunking the myths that have surrounded the word "fat" for years.

Eating Fat Makes You Fat

On the surface, the theory that eating fat makes you fat seems like a no-brainer. Of the three macronutrients—protein, carbohydrates, and fat—fat contains the most calories per gram. Protein and carbohydrates have 4 calories per gram, while fat contains more than twice that at 9 calories per gram. It would make sense that if you cut out fat or replace fat with protein or carbohydrates at each meal, you would be saving yourself a ton of calories throughout the course of the day. While technically you would save on calories, it doesn't lead to sustainable weight loss.

 Fact

As the low-fat diet gained in popularity, there was also an increase in the availability of low-fat food items, such as cookies and candy bars. To create these items, manufacturers removed fat and replaced it with sugar to keep it palatable so consumers would continue to buy the product. These packaged food items were lower in fat, but they were higher in sugar and contained the same, if not more, calories.

In order to understand why fat doesn't make you fat, you have to understand how you gain weight in the first place. The simple explanation is this: You start thinking about food and your body secretes insulin in response. The insulin triggers a response that tells your body to store fatty acids instead of using them for energy, so you get hungry. When you get hungry, you eat. If you're on a low-fat diet, your lunch may consist of two slices of whole-wheat toast with a couple of slices of turkey—no cheese, no mayo—and an apple on the side. If you've subscribed to the low-fat diet theory, this seems like a healthy meal, but in reality, it's loaded with carbohydrates that pass through your digestive system quickly, causing significant spikes in blood sugar, and has virtually no fat.

Your body quickly breaks down your high-carbohydrate meal, which sends a rush of glucose into your bloodstream. Your body responds to this glucose by secreting more insulin, which carries the glucose out of your blood and into your cells. Once the glucose levels drop, you get hungry again, your body secretes more insulin, and the cycle starts over.

 Essential

Carbohydrates are a fast-acting source of energy for your body, but they don't do a lot to fill you up. Even carbohydrates that are loaded with fiber are far less satiating than either protein or fat. If you want your meal to be truly satisfying, make sure it contains plenty of fat.

Here's where you'll want to pay close attention. Your body's main regulator of fat metabolism is insulin. Insulin controls lipoprotein lipase, or LPL, an enzyme that pulls fat into your cells. The higher your insulin levels, the more fat LPL pulls into your cells. Translation: when insulin levels increase, you store fat. When insulin levels drop, you burn fat for energy. The main thing that affects insulin levels is carbohydrates, not fat. So when you eat a lot of carbohydrates, your insulin levels increase, which increases your LPL levels, which increases your storage of fat.

It's important to remember that overdoing it on any of the nutrients will lead to weight gain. Regularly exceeding your caloric needs will cause weight gain regardless of whether you do it with carbohydrates, protein, or fat—but fat is not the major culprit when it comes to weight gain.

Cholesterol Causes Heart Disease

The cholesterol you eat actually has very little impact on your blood cholesterol levels for two reasons. The first reason is that your body doesn't absorb dietary cholesterol very efficiently. Most of the cholesterol you eat goes right through your digestive tract and never even enters your bloodstream. The second reason is that the amount of cholesterol in your blood is tightly controlled by your body. When you eat a lot of dietary cholesterol, your body shuts down its own production of cholesterol to compensate. There is a percentage of the population, however, that is hypersensitive to dietary cholesterol. For these people—about 25 percent of the population—dietary cholesterol does cause modest increases in both LDL (low-density lipoprotein) and HDL (high-density lipoprotein) levels, but even so, the increased cholesterol levels do not increase the risk of heart disease. In fact, both the Framingham Heart Study and the Honolulu Heart Program found the opposite to be true: Low cholesterol levels were actually associated with increased risk of death. A separate study published in the *Journal of the American Medical Association* reported findings that neither high LDL ("bad" cholesterol) levels nor low HDL ("good" cholesterol) levels were important risk factors for death from coronary artery disease or heart attack.

 Fact

Most of the cholesterol in your blood (75 percent) is actually made in your body. Only 25 percent comes from the food you eat. If you followed a completely cholesterol-free diet, your body would compensate by increasing its cholesterol production by the liver to keep your blood levels steady. That's because your body needs cholesterol to survive.

Cholesterol is absolutely essential for your survival. This lipoprotein, as it is physiologically classified, performs three major functions. It makes up the bile acids that help you digest food, it allows the body to make vitamin D and other essential hormones such as estrogen and testosterone, and it is a component of the outer coating of every one of your cells. Without cholesterol, your body would literally crumble.

That's not to say that you should throw all caution out the window when it comes to cholesterol, but you need to pay attention to the right thing, and that's the size of the cholesterol particles in your bloodstream rather than the total numbers. Cholesterol comes in two forms: large particles that "bounce" off the arterial walls and small, dense particles that stick to the walls of your arteries and contribute to arterial blockage, which can eventually lead to heart disease. The problem is that so much focus is placed on the total numbers that many people fail to pay attention to cholesterol particle size.

 Alert

The focus has been so much on high cholesterol that doctors seem to have forgotten the risks associated with low cholesterol levels. Without sufficient cholesterol your immune system cannot properly function, you cannot produce sufficient steroid hormones (leading to severe sex hormone imbalances), your cell membranes get weak, and you end up with impaired memory and brain function.

According to Dr. Mark Hyman, a functional medicine doctor at the UltraWellness Center in Lenox, Massachusetts, it's not fat that causes the accumulation of small, dense cholesterol particles in your blood; it's sugar. And that's sugar in any form, including refined carbohydrates. Sugar decreases the amount of the large cholesterol particles in your blood, creates the small damaging cholesterol particles, increases triglyceride levels, and contributes to prediabetes.

Saturated Fat Causes Heart Disease
The other widespread belief is that eating saturated fat causes an increase in the amount of cholesterol in your blood, which in turn causes heart disease or increases your risk of heart disease. This theory was developed from some human and animal studies that were done decades ago. However, more recent research calls this theory into question.

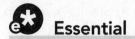 **Essential**

The idea that eating cholesterol causes heart disease is called the diet-heart hypothesis. The theory that high cholesterol levels in the blood cause heart disease is called the lipid hypothesis. Both of these hypotheses are so widely accepted that most healthcare professionals and consumers don't even question them, although more recent research has shown that cholesterol and heart disease may not be as interconnected as previously believed. Inflammation, especially low-grade chronic inflammation driven by excess carbohydrate consumption, has been found to be the real driver of cardiovascular disease.

In 2010, the *American Journal of Clinical Nutrition* did a meta-analysis of several studies that investigated the relationship between saturated fat and heart disease and concluded that there is no significant evidence to make the claim that dietary saturated fat is associated with increased risk of coronary heart disease or cardiovascular disease, in general. In fact, several of the studies the journal investigated showed a positive inverse relationship, which means that a higher intake of saturated fat was actually associated with a lower incidence of heart disease.

Why Fat Is Your Friend

Fat is an integral part of every cell in your body. This macronutrient is a major component of your cell membranes, which hold each cell together. Every single cell in your body, from the cells in your brain to the cells in your heart to the cells in your lungs, is dependent on fat for survival. Fat is especially important for your brain, which is made up of 60 percent fat and cholesterol.

Fat and cholesterol are used as building blocks for many hormones, which help regulate metabolism, control growth and development, and maintain bone and muscle mass, among many other things. Fat is vital for proper immune function, helps regulate body temperature, and serves as a source of protection for your major organs. Fat surrounds all of your vital organs to provide a sort of cushion for protection against falls and trauma. Fat also helps boost metabolic function and plays a role in keeping you lean.

Fat is an essential nutrient. This means that you need to ingest it through the foods you eat because the body cannot make what it needs on its own. Fat is composed of individual molecules called fatty acids. Two of these fatty acids, omega-3 fatty acids and omega-6 fatty acids, are absolutely essential for good health. Omega-3 fatty acids play a crucial role in brain function and growth and development, while omega-6 fatty acids help regulate metabolism and maintain bone health. Fat also allows you to absorb and digest other essential nutrients, such as vitamins A, D, E, and K, and beta carotene. Without enough fat in your diet, you wouldn't be able to absorb any of these nutrients and you would eventually develop nutritional deficiencies.

As if that weren't enough, fat is a major source of energy for your body. The fact that each gram of fat contains 9 calories is actually a good thing. This makes it a compact source of energy that your body can use easily and efficiently. Unlike with carbohydrates, which your body can only store in limited amounts, your body has an unlimited ability to store fat for later use. When food intake falls short, as between meals or while you're sleeping, your body calls on its fat reservoirs for energy. This physiological process is what the entire ketogenic diet is based on.

Your body needs a continuous source of energy to maintain its functions. The body's preferred source of energy, because it's fast acting and easily accessible, is glucose, which comes from carbohydrates. When you give your body access to glucose, it stores fat in your fat cells for later use. When you deprive the body of glucose, it turns to fat for energy.

Reducing Body Fat

Now that you know what causes your body to store fat, the obvious next question is, how do you use that knowledge to help reduce your body fat? The quick answer, and one that may seem counter-intuitive at this point, is to eat more fat, but it's not that simple. You can't simply add fat to a diet that's full of carbohydrates and loaded with protein and expect the weight to fall off. You need to reduce carbohydrates in order to achieve a state of ketosis and maximize the fat-burning ability of the body, and get to that stored body fat. In other words: a ketogenic diet.

 Fact

Researchers at the Karolinska Institutet, in Stockholm, Sweden, found that the number of fat cells you have as an adult remains the same no matter how much weight you lose. When you lose weight, the number of fat cells doesn't actually decrease; the cells just shrink in size, essentially taking up less room and making you look leaner.

The Importance of a Healthy Body-Fat Level

Fat is important, there's no doubt about that, but too much on your body can be bad for your health. Having excess body fat increases your risk of various health problems, including:

- Type 2 diabetes
- Heart disease
- Gallstones
- Sleep apnea
- Certain types of cancers
- High blood pressure
- Stroke
- Osteoarthritis
- Fatty liver disease
- Infertility
- Kidney disease
- Gestational diabetes

Reducing the amount of fat you carry on your body can help reduce your risk of developing these chronic conditions, even if you have a family history of them.

Improving Your Blood Sugar
and Insulin Levels

A major component to keeping yourself healthy, or improving any current health problems, is regulating your blood sugar and insulin levels. Imbalances in blood sugar and insulin are significant factors in the rapidly growing epidemic in diabetes in both children and adults.

Insulin Resistance and Diabetes

You already know that insulin is responsible for bringing the glucose from your bloodstream into your cells so that your body can use it as energy, but insulin also stimulates your liver and muscles to store excess glucose, which is called glycogen, for later use. In a healthy person, insulin and glucose do their jobs effectively and efficiently, and as a result, both insulin and glucose levels remain within a certain healthy range.

 Alert

Many people aren't aware that they have insulin resistance until they are officially diagnosed with prediabetes or type 2 diabetes. Early warning signs of insulin resistance include fatigue, energy crashes, carbohydrate cravings, and weight gain around the midsection. If you experience any of these warning signs, it may be beneficial to have your insulin and glucose levels tested.

Insulin resistance is a condition in which the pancreas produces enough insulin, but the body is not able to use it effectively. When you're repeatedly exposed to high levels of insulin, your cells begin to say, "No, thank you" and start building up a resistance to insulin. When insulin, which carries glucose on its back, can't enter the cells, glucose remains in the bloodstream as well. This signals the pancreas to release even more insulin, which only exacerbates the cycle. While your body may be able to sustain this added stress for a certain period of time, eventually the pancreas gives up and insulin production decreases or stops altogether.

Without insulin, glucose can't enter the cells, so it stays in the bloodstream, wreaking havoc on your system. This is the point when many people are diagnosed with prediabetes or type 2 diabetes. Elevated glucose levels also contribute to obesity, high blood pressure, heart disease, certain types of cancer, and neurodegenerative disorders such as Alzheimer's disease.

What Do Carbs Do?

When you eat carbohydrates, your body breaks them down into glucose. The rate at which this happens differs depending on the type of carbohydrates you're eating, but eventually, all carbohydrates, with the exception of fiber, become glucose. When glucose enters your bloodstream, it triggers the release of insulin, as you already know. Constantly bombarding your body with carbohydrates and refined sugars increases glucose and insulin levels dramatically, increasing your risk of developing insulin resistance and the other resulting health problems. The goal is to avoid surges and crashes in glucose and insulin and to keep your levels consistent and steady throughout the day. When you do this, your body is better able to handle both glucose and insulin over the long term.

How Fat Can Help

Unlike carbohydrates and refined sugars, eating fat doesn't cause a dramatic spike in glucose or insulin levels. When you turn your body from burning glucose for fuel to burning fat for fuel, which is the basis of the ketogenic diet, you help stabilize your glucose and insulin levels, which decreases your chances of developing insulin resistance.

Feeling Satisfied While Losing Weight

One of the biggest complaints you'll hear from dieters on a weight-loss program is that they don't feel satisfied. They're always hungry or the food just isn't good. This is where most diets fail. If you're always hungry on a diet, what are the chances that you're going to be able to stick to it long-term? Probably close to zero. No one wants to be hungry all the time. On the other hand, consistently eating foods that lack any flavor and always leave you wanting more is a recipe for disaster. At some point, your cravings for delicious, satiating foods are going to triumph over your determination to lose weight and you're going to give in to temptation—and probably in a big way. Feelings of deprivation are one of the biggest causes of eventual binges. This is where fat shines.

 Fact

Foods with a high fat content tend to taste so good because many different flavors dissolve in fats. Butter especially works as an excellent carrier for a wide variety of flavors, including spices, vanilla, and other fat-soluble ingredients. The human body is also genetically programmed to seek out high-energy foods. Because of this, fatty foods are inherently perceived as more flavorful.

When you cut fat out of your diet, it's hard to reach that point when you really feel satisfied. This is why people on low-fat diets complain of being hungry all the time. Fat also adds a ton of flavor to food, so when you eat fat you're actually enjoying the food you're eating, which makes you more likely to stick to your diet plan. Sounds like a no-brainer, right?

What Are Fat Bombs?

Fat bombs are low-carbohydrate, high-fat recipes or foods that include a high percentage of fat and a low percentage of carbohydrates. Fat bombs were originally created as pure fat snacks to reach your fat macronutrient goal for the day when following a ketogenic diet. Since the ketogenic diet requires such high levels of fat for the body to enter and stay in ketosis, fat bombs are an easy solution to help dieters reach their fat requirements each day. Over time, and with the widespread use of the diet, the concept of the fat bomb has widened a little to include small meals with an adequate ratio of protein to fat that also keep the carbohydrate content to a minimum. These snacks and meals, when consumed throughout the day, will help you successfully maintain your macronutrient ratios for the diet while providing necessary nutrients and keeping you satisfied.

Adapting to a High-Fat Diet

The concept of a "fat bomb" can be quite shocking if you are not familiar with the principles and challenges of a ketogenic diet. At first a fat bomb may sound quite unappealing to you, but once you understand its value and application within the diet, you will be eager to try all the enticing and flavorful ways to get more fat into your body.

One of the hardest parts of the ketogenic diet is matching your required fat intake, especially at the beginning. If you are transitioning from a long-term, low-fat dieting plan, chances are, you forgot how to use fats in your diet.

Current low-fat recipe trends combined with ready-made "healthy" meals sold in supermarkets will not help you meet your weight-loss or health goals. Often they are high in carbohydrates and sugar, despite being labeled as "healthy" because they are low in fat. Once you start keeping track of your macros on a ketogenic diet, you'll find yourself reaching your carbohydrate limit early in the day, while you still have a lot of calories left to fill in the form of fat and protein. The fat bomb is the easy solution for this seemingly impossible problem.

Using Fat Bombs for Success on the Ketogenic Diet

Fat bombs can be used to balance your macronutrient intake of fat and protein while leaving your carbohydrate intake adequately low. You can start your day with a savory, egg-based fat bomb for breakfast to get a head start in consuming healthy fats and make sure your blood sugar will be stable for the rest of the day. Or, you can add in a fat-bomb snack in the middle of your day to combat that mid-afternoon slump and problematic sugar craving. Another idea is to use a small fat-bomb dinner to keep your caloric intake as low as needed and fill your need for fat. These are just some of the ways a fat bomb can be your invaluable ally for your success with a ketogenic diet.

Using Savory Fat Bombs

Many fat-bomb recipes feature sweet ingredients to make the fats more palatable. However, as you adjust to adding fat bombs to your diet, you'll need to balance savory with sweet. In addition to the benefits of savory fat bombs as meal replacers, there is another very important reason to use savory, instead of just eating the sweet, "treat-like" ones. Sugar consumption is directly related to insulin release into the bloodstream. Your body becomes so trained to expect a blood sugar spike following the ingestion of sweet-flavored foods that it creates an almost automatic response. It is clinically proven that the ingestion of noncalorie sweeteners will still trigger an insulin response in the body, especially if you are insulin resistant. That mechanism is proven by the fact that a sweet-flavored treat with the same macronutrient ratios as a savory one will make you hungry much sooner. When weaning yourself from the habit of sugar, the sweet flavor alone can become a trigger for powerful cravings, even if the sweetener had zero carbohydrates in it.

Enjoying Liquid Fat Bombs

Convenience will make it easier to successfully stick to your eating plan. Liquid fat bombs are a great way to help you get the right balance of fats, proteins, and carbohydrates for your body. When pressed for time it can be invaluable to be able to throw a few ingredients into a blender and make it a meal. Liquid fat bombs can be easily created, easily transported, and easily shared. They will provide the right macronutrients your body needs, some essential nutrients, and a lot of great flavor to your diet.

CHAPTER 4

Balls

Avocado, Macadamia, and Prosciutto Balls DF

The subtle, smooth flavors of avocado and macadamia nuts make a perfect counterpoint for salty prosciutto and spicy pepper.

Prep Time: 7 minutes • Cook Time: 0 minutes

MAKES 6 FAT BOMBS

4 ounces macadamia nuts

4 ounces (½ large) avocado pulp

1 ounce cooked prosciutto, crumbled (for cooking instructions see Appendix A)

¼ teaspoon freshly ground black pepper

1. In a small food processor, pulse macadamia nuts until evenly crumbled. Divide in half.
2. In a small bowl, combine avocado, half the macadamia nuts, prosciutto crumbles, and pepper and mix well with a fork.
3. Form mixture into 6 balls.
4. Place remaining crumbled macadamia nuts on a medium plate and roll individual balls through to coat evenly.
5. Serve immediately.

PER 1 FAT BOMB Calories: 170 | Fat: 17g | Protein: 3g | Sodium: 44mg | Fiber: 3g | Carbohydrates: 5g | Sugar: 1g

Bacon Jalapeño Balls

Enjoy a little kick of fire in these Mexican-flavored fat bombs.

Prep Time: 10 minutes • Cook Time: 0 minutes

MAKES 6 FAT BOMBS

3 ounces cooked bacon, fat reserved
3 ounces cream cheese
2 tablespoons reserved bacon fat
1 teaspoon seeded and finely chopped jalapeño pepper
1 tablespoon finely chopped cilantro

1. On a cutting board, chop bacon into small crumbs.
2. In a small bowl, combine cream cheese, bacon fat, jalapeño, and cilantro; mix well with a fork.
3. Form mixture into 6 balls.
4. Place bacon crumbles on a medium plate and roll individual balls through to coat evenly.
5. Serve immediately or refrigerate up to 3 days.

PER 1 FAT BOMB Calories: 135 | Fat: 11g | Protein: 7g | Sodium: 408mg | Fiber: 0g | Carbohydrates: 1g | Sugar: 0g

Bacon Maple Pancake Balls

These fat bombs have the flavor of breakfast pancakes with maple syrup and bacon. They're a great way to start the day off right!

Prep Time: 10 minutes • Cook Time: 0 minutes

MAKES 6 FAT BOMBS

3 ounces cooked bacon

3 ounces cream cheese

½ teaspoon maple flavor

¼ teaspoon salt

3 tablespoons crushed pecans

1. On a cutting board, chop bacon into small crumbs.
2. In a small bowl, combine cream cheese and bacon crumbles with maple flavor and salt; mix well with a fork.
3. Form mixture into 6 balls.
4. Place crushed pecans on a medium plate and roll individual balls through to coat evenly.
5. Serve immediately or refrigerate up to 3 days.

> **Food Flavoring versus Sugar-Free Syrup**
>
> A lot of recipes on the ketogenic diet call for sugar-free syrup. Such syrups contain ingredients like acesulfame potassium, sodium hexametaphosphate, or phosphoric acid. Those artificial flavors, preservatives, and fillers are not health-building ingredients; on the contrary, they load the body with toxins, which make it much harder to lose unwanted pounds. A good organic maple flavor will only contain a maple distillate and pure grain alcohol in minimal quantities.

PER 1 FAT BOMB Calories: 148 | Fat: 13g | Protein: 6g | Sodium: 467mg | Fiber: 0g | Carbohydrates: 1g | Sugar: 1g

Barbecue Balls

An easy way to get your barbecue fix—and your fat too. You will be surprised how much these fat bombs taste like barbecue sauce.

Prep Time: 2 hours 5 minutes • Cook Time: 0 minutes

MAKES 6 FAT BOMBS

4 ounces cream cheese
4 tablespoons bacon fat
½ teaspoon smoke flavor
2 drops stevia glycerite
⅛ teaspoon apple cider vinegar
1 tablespoon sweet smoked chili powder

1. In a small food processor, process all ingredients except chili powder until they form a smooth cream, about 30 seconds.
2. Scrape mixture and transfer into a small bowl, then refrigerate 2 hours.
3. Form into 6 balls with the aid of a spoon.
4. Sprinkle balls with chili powder, rolling around to coat all sides.
5. Serve immediately or refrigerate up to 3 days.

PER 1 FAT BOMB Calories: 154 | Fat: 13g | Protein: 3g | Sodium: 186mg | Fiber: 0g | Carbohydrates: 1g | Sugar: 1g

Kalamata Olive and Feta Balls

This recipe brings you the flavors of Greece on a warm sunny day by the Mediterranean Sea.

Prep Time: 2 hours 5 minutes • Cook Time: 0 minutes

MAKES 6 FAT BOMBS

2 ounces cream cheese
2 ounces feta
12 large kalamata olives, pitted

⅛ teaspoon finely chopped fresh thyme
⅛ teaspoon fresh lemon zest

1. In a small food processor, process all ingredients until they form a coarse dough, about 30 seconds.
2. Scrape mixture and transfer to a small bowl, then refrigerate 2 hours.
3. Form into 6 balls with the aid of a spoon.
4. Serve immediately or refrigerate up to 3 days.

PER 1 FAT BOMB Calories: 61 | Fat: 5g | Protein: 2g | Sodium: 135mg | Fiber: 0g | Carbohydrates: 2g | Sugar: 1g

Brie Hazelnut Balls

This is another super-easy fat-bomb recipe, bursting with delicious flavor. The warm notes of toasted hazelnuts and fresh flavor of thyme really brighten the soft flavor of Brie.

Prep Time: 2 hours 5 minutes • Cook Time: 0 minutes

MAKES 6 FAT BOMBS

4 ounces Brie
2 ounces toasted hazelnuts

⅛ teaspoon finely chopped fresh thyme

1. In a small food processor, process all ingredients until they form a coarse dough, about 30 seconds.
2. Scrape mixture and transfer to a small bowl and refrigerate 2 hours.
3. Form into 6 balls with the aid of a spoon.
4. Serve immediately or refrigerate up to 3 days.

PER 1 FAT BOMB Calories: 121 | Fat: 11g | Protein: 5g | Sodium: 117mg | Fiber: 1g | Carbohydrates: 2g | Sugar: 0g

Carbonara Balls

Do you like Italian food and have a craving for spaghetti carbonara? This is the fat-bomb version of that fantastic recipe.

Prep Time: 8 minutes • Cook Time: 0 minutes

MAKES 6 FAT BOMBS

3 ounces cooked bacon

3 ounces mascarpone

2 large hard-boiled egg yolks

¼ teaspoon freshly ground black pepper

1. On a cutting board, chop bacon into small crumbs.
2. In a small bowl, combine mascarpone, egg yolks, and pepper; mix well with a fork.
3. Form mascarpone mixture into 6 balls.
4. Place bacon crumbles on a medium plate and roll individual balls through to coat evenly.
5. Serve immediately or refrigerate up to 3 days.

PER 1 FAT BOMB Calories: 148 | Fat: 12g | Protein: 8g | Sodium: 392mg | Fiber: 0g | Carbohydrates: 1g | Sugar: 1g

Two Different Ways to Cook Bacon

There are two different ways you can get your bacon ready for this recipe or any other recipe in this book. For the pan-frying method: Place the bacon slices closely together in a cold frying pan. Cook over medium heat without moving the slices for about 5 minutes. The bacon should by then move easily and not be stuck to the bottom of the pan. Flip the bacon and cook for about 5 more minutes. Remove from the pan and drain on a paper towel. For the oven method: Preheat oven to 400°F. Place a rack on a baking sheet. Lay the bacon slices on the rack and bake for 10–15 minutes depending on desired doneness level.

Creamy and Crunchy Egg Balls

These fat bombs are a delightful combination of soft, creamy, and crunchy textures, and savory, salty flavors.

Prep Time: 40 minutes • Cook Time: 0 minutes

MAKES 6 FAT BOMBS

2 medium eggs, hard-boiled and peeled
2 tablespoons cream cheese
1 tablespoon coconut oil, melted
2 slices prosciutto, cooked and crumbled

1. Place eggs, cream cheese, and coconut oil in a food processor and pulse until well mixed.
2. Place food processor bowl in refrigerator a minimum 30 minutes or until mixture solidifies.
3. Once egg mixture is solid, remove from refrigerator and shape into 6 balls with the aid of a spoon.
4. Place prosciutto crumbles on a medium plate and roll individual balls through to coat.
5. Serve immediately or refrigerate in an airtight container up to 4 days.

PER 1 FAT BOMB Calories: 67 | Fat: 6g | Protein: 4g |
Sodium: 131mg | Fiber: 0g | Carbohydrates: 0g | Sugar: 0g

Creamy Olive Balls

The sharp and tangy flavor of kalamata olives combines beautifully with the creaminess of cheese in this recipe.

Prep Time: 40 minutes • Cook Time: 0 minutes

MAKES 6 FAT BOMBS

6 large kalamata olives, pitted
2 tablespoons cream cheese
1 tablespoon coconut oil, melted
2 tablespoons hemp hearts

> **Hemp Hearts**
> Hemp hearts are the shelled seeds of the hemp plant. They do not contain any psychoactive compounds, but they do contain a lot of great omega-3s. They are becoming more and more popular because of their great nutrient content and sustainable origin. They have great macros for a fat bomb: Per 30-gram serving, hemp hearts contain 10 grams of plant-based protein and 10 grams of omega-3s.

1. Place olives, cream cheese, and coconut oil in a food processor and pulse until very well mixed.
2. Place food processor bowl in refrigerator a minimum 30 minutes or until mixture solidifies.
3. Once mixture is solid, remove from refrigerator and shape into 6 balls with the aid of a spoon.
4. Place hemp hearts on a medium plate and roll individual balls through to coat.
5. Serve immediately or refrigerate in an airtight container up to 4 days.

PER 1 FAT BOMB Calories: 71 | Fat: 4g | Protein: 3g | Sodium: 18mg | Fiber: 0g | Carbohydrates: 6g | Sugar: 2g

Curried Tuna Balls

Just a touch of spice gives this recipe a different twist on the usual fat bomb. It's enough to keep your taste buds entertained and satisfied.

Prep Time: 10 minutes • Cook Time: 0 minutes

MAKES 6 FAT BOMBS

3 ounces tuna in oil, drained

2 ounces cream cheese

¼ teaspoon curry powder, divided

1 ounce crumbled macadamia nuts

Mercury Concerns

If you're concerned about the mercury in tuna, keep in mind that adults can safely eat 18–24 ounces of tuna per month without a significant amount of mercury getting into their systems. If you'd like, swap out the tuna for canned salmon. Canned salmon is higher in omega-3 fatty acids and contains lower levels of mercury.

1. In a small food processor, process tuna, cream cheese, and half the curry powder until they form a smooth cream, about 30 seconds.
2. Form mixture into 6 balls.
3. Place crumbled macadamia nuts and remaining curry powder on a medium plate and roll individual balls through to coat evenly.
4. Serve immediately or refrigerate up to 3 days.

PER 1 FAT BOMB Calories: 93 | Fat: 8g | Protein: 5g | Sodium: 80mg | Fiber: 0g | Carbohydrates: 1g | Sugar: 1g

Egg Tapenade Balls DF

You may have used chia seeds before, but they were probably soaked in some liquid! You will be surprised at how well they work as a coating element. They're a little crunchy with mild flavor and have a perfect nutritional profile!

Prep Time: 40 minutes • Cook Time: 0 minutes

MAKES 6 FAT BOMBS

2 medium hard-boiled eggs, peeled
6 large kalamata olives, pitted
1 anchovy fillet
1 tablespoon coconut oil, melted
2 tablespoons chia seeds

> **A Fancy French Word**
> *Tapenade* is a fancy French word for a basic olive spread usually consisting of olives, capers, and anchovies. Anchovies provide great flavor and healthy omega-3s. You can always skip them if you do not enjoy the flavor.

1. Place eggs, olives, anchovy fillet, and coconut oil in a food processor and pulse until mixed but not overblended.
2. Place food processor bowl in refrigerator a minimum 30 minutes or until mixture solidifies.
3. Once egg mixture is solid, remove from refrigerator and shape into 6 balls with the aid of a spoon.
4. Place chia seeds on a medium plate and roll individual balls through to coat.
5. Serve immediately or refrigerate in an airtight container up to 4 days.

PER 1 FAT BOMB Calories: 86 | Fat: 6g | Protein: 5g | Sodium: 298mg | Fiber: 1g | Carbohydrates: 5g | Sugar: 0g

For the Love of Pork Bombs

Any day with bacon is a great day. Add liverwurst, pistachios, and cream cheese, and the flavors become a symphony of perfect pork cuisine for any true bacon lover!

Prep Time: 1 hour 15 minutes • Cook Time: 10 minutes

MAKES 12 FAT BOMBS

8 slices bacon

8 ounces Braunschweiger, at room temperature

¼ cup chopped pistachios

6 ounces cream cheese, at room temperature

1 teaspoon Dijon mustard

> **Is Braunschweiger the Same as Liverwurst?**
> While the ingredients in both sausages are similar (pork and pork liver), many times Braunschweiger also contains bacon. Braunschweiger is generally soft and spreadable, whereas liverwurst is firmer and better for slicing.

1. Cook bacon in a medium skillet over medium heat until crisp, 5 minutes per side. Drain on paper towels and let cool. Once cooled, crumble into bacon-bit-sized pieces.

2. Place Braunschweiger with pistachios in a small food processor and pulse until just combined.

3. In a small mixing bowl, use a hand blender to whip cream cheese and Dijon mustard until combined and fluffy.

4. Divide meat mixture into 12 equal servings. Roll into balls and cover in a thin layer of cream cheese mixture.

5. Chill at least 1 hour. When ready to serve, place bacon bits on a medium plate, roll balls through to coat evenly, and enjoy.

6. Fat bombs can be refrigerated in an airtight container up to 4 days.

PER 1 FAT BOMB Calories: 192 | Fat: 18g | Protein: 6g | Sodium: 392mg | Fiber: 0g | Carbohydrates: 2g | Sugar: 1g

Pizza Balls

This recipe takes the ultimate Italian dish and magically transforms it into a fat bomb. Whenever the urge for pizza hits you, reach for this instead.

Prep Time: 8 minutes • Cook Time: 0 minutes

MAKES 6 FAT BOMBS

2 ounces fresh mozzarella

2 ounces cream cheese

1 tablespoon olive oil

1 teaspoon tomato paste

6 large kalamata olives, pitted

12 fresh basil leaves

1. In a small food processor, process all ingredients except basil until they form a smooth cream, about 30 seconds.
2. Form mixture into 6 balls with the aid of a spoon.
3. Place 1 basil leaf on top and bottom of each ball and secure with a toothpick.
4. Serve immediately or refrigerate up to 3 days.

PER 1 FAT BOMB Calories: 82 | Fat: 8g | Protein: 3g | Sodium: 96mg | Fiber: 0g | Carbohydrates: 1g | Sugar: 1g

Salted Caramel and Brie Balls

You will love this super-easy and fast recipe. It features three ingredients and takes under 5 minutes to make.

Prep Time: 5 minutes • Cook Time: 0 minutes

MAKES 6 FAT BOMBS

4 ounces roughly chopped Brie

2 ounces salted macadamia nuts

½ teaspoon caramel flavor

1. In a small food processor, process all ingredients until they form a coarse dough, about 30 seconds.
2. Form mixture into 6 balls with the aid of a spoon.
3. Serve immediately or refrigerate up to 3 days.

PER 1 FAT BOMB Calories: 130 | Fat: 12g | Protein: 5g | Sodium: 118mg | Fiber: 1g | Carbohydrates: 1g | Sugar: 1g

Prosciutto and Egg Balls DF

This is another dairy-free fat bomb. The coconut oil provides a great source of good fats and is casein- and lactose-free, suitable for people with dairy intolerances. It also helps the fat bomb stick together without changing the flavor.

Prep Time: 40 minutes • Cook Time: 0 minutes

MAKES 6 FAT BOMBS

2 medium hard-boiled eggs, peeled

2 tablespoons mayonnaise

⅛ teaspoon freshly ground black pepper

⅛ teaspoon sea salt

1 tablespoon coconut oil, melted

2 slices prosciutto, cooked and crumbled (see sidebar)

> **Prosciutto Crumbles**
>
> To make easy prosciutto crumbles, simply bake them in the oven. Preheat oven to 350°F. Place the thin prosciutto slices on a cookie sheet and bake them for about 12 minutes. Remove from the oven and let cool. Once cold and crispy, chop finely with a sharp kitchen knife until reduced to crumbles.

1. Place eggs, mayonnaise, pepper, and salt in a small bowl. Mash with a fork to mix and combine while still retaining some texture.
2. Pour melted coconut oil into mixture and blend in well.
3. Place bowl in refrigerator a minimum 30 minutes or until mixture solidifies.
4. Once egg mixture is solid, remove from refrigerator and shape into 6 balls with the aid of a spoon.
5. Place prosciutto crumbles on a medium plate and roll individual balls through to coat.
6. Serve immediately or refrigerate in an airtight container up to 4 days.

PER 1 FAT BOMB Calories: 84 | Fat: 8g | Protein: 4g | Sodium: 191mg | Fiber: 0g | Carbohydrates: 0g | Sugar: 0g

Salmon Mascarpone Balls

Omega-3s are essential fatty acids, which means your body cannot manufacture them and must get them from your diet. This recipe is not only rich in beneficial omega-3s, but it also has a creamy, smooth mouthfeel.

Prep Time: 7 minutes • Cook Time: 0 minutes

MAKES 6 FAT BOMBS

3 ounces smoked salmon, chopped

3 ounces mascarpone

½ teaspoon maple flavor

½ teaspoon chopped chives

3 tablespoons hemp hearts

> **Smoked Salmon**
> When buying smoked salmon, please make sure you get either wild or sustainably farmed. Often, conventionally farmed salmon contains high levels of antibiotics. Antibiotics from industrially farmed animals contribute to the creation of antibiotic-resistant superbugs.

1. In a small food processor, combine salmon, mascarpone, maple flavor, and chives. Pulse a few times until blended together.
2. Form mixture into 6 balls.
3. Put hemp hearts on a medium plate and roll individual balls through to coat evenly.
4. Serve immediately or refrigerate up to 3 days.

PER 1 FAT BOMB Calories: 65 | Fat: 5g | Protein: 3g | Sodium: 155mg | Fiber: 0g | Carbohydrates: 1g | Sugar: 0g

Spicy Bacon and Avocado Balls DF

These fat bombs carry some of the flavors of guacamole. They are slightly spicy, but if you want to increase the fire, just leave some of the jalapeño seeds in.

Prep Time: 45 minutes • Cook Time: 8 minutes

MAKES 6 FAT BOMBS

4 slices bacon

1 medium avocado, pitted and peeled

2 tablespoons coconut oil

1 tablespoon bacon fat

1 tablespoon finely chopped green onions

2 tablespoons finely chopped cilantro

1 small jalapeño pepper, seeded and finely chopped

¼ teaspoon sea salt

> **Hot Jalapeños**
>
> Jalapeño peppers can vary greatly in their degree of heat. In the same batch you can find quite mild ones and some very spicy ones. Even if you like it hot, start your recipes without the seeds . . . you can always add heat, but you can't remove it!

1. In a medium nonstick skillet over medium heat, cook bacon until golden, about 4 minutes each side.
2. Drain bacon on a paper towel. Save bacon fat for later in a glass cup.
3. Once bacon is cool, chop 2 slices into crumbles.
4. Cut remaining 2 slices into 3 pieces each; these will be the bases for your fat bombs.
5. Smash avocado with a fork in a small bowl.
6. Add coconut oil and cooled bacon fat to avocado.
7. Add onion, cilantro, jalapeño, salt, and bacon crumbles. Blend well with a fork.
8. Refrigerate a minimum 30 minutes.
9. Form mixture into 6 balls with the aid of a spoon.
10. Place remaining 6 bacon pieces on a plate, then top each with an avocado ball.
11. Serve immediately or refrigerate up to 3 days.

PER 1 FAT BOMB Calories: 181 | Fat: 18g | Protein: 3g | Sodium: 258mg | Fiber: 2g | Carbohydrates: 3g | Sugar: 0g

Sunbutter Balls

This recipe could also be called the Cravings Killer, as it can help to curb your sugar cravings naturally!

Prep Time: 20 minutes • Cook Time: 0 minutes

MAKES 12 FAT BOMBS

6 tablespoons mascarpone

3 tablespoons sunflower seed butter

6 tablespoons coconut oil, softened

3 tablespoons unsweetened shredded coconut flakes

> ### An Italian Delight
> Mascarpone is an Italian soft cheese best known for being used in the famous tiramisu. It is actually the perfect ingredient for fat bombs; it's creamy, delicious, and contains zero carbs!

1. In a medium bowl, mix mascarpone, sunflower seed butter, and coconut oil until a smooth paste forms.
2. Shape paste into walnut-sized balls. If mixture is too sticky, place in refrigerator 15 minutes before forming balls.
3. Spread coconut flakes on a medium plate and roll individual balls through to coat evenly.

PER 1 FAT BOMB Calories: 124 | Fat: 13g | Protein: 2g | Sodium: 43mg | Fiber: 1g | Carbohydrates: 2g | Sugar: 1g

CHAPTER 5

Chicken Skin Crisps

Chicken Skin Crisps Alfredo

Alfredo sauce must be one of the most well-loved sauces for both chicken and noodles. Here you can get all the flavor of Alfredo sauce without any of the carbs usually involved!

Prep Time: 5 minutes • Cook Time: 20 minutes

MAKES 6 FAT BOMBS
Skin from 3 chicken thighs
2 tablespoons ricotta
2 tablespoons cream cheese
1 tablespoon grated Parmesan
¼ garlic clove, minced
¼ teaspoon ground white pepper

> **Chicken Skin Crisps**
> You can either buy chicken thighs and remove the skin to make your chicken skin crisps, or you can ask your local butcher or farmer from the farmers' market to sell you just chicken skin. You will be surprised; chicken skin is not so hard to find, and it will make superb crisps to use instead of crackers.

1. Preheat oven to 350°F. On a cookie sheet, lay out skins as flat as possible.
2. Bake 12–15 minutes until skins turn light brown and crispy being careful not to burn them.
3. Remove skins from cookie sheet and place on a paper towel to cool.
4. In a small bowl, add cheeses, garlic, and pepper. Mix with a fork until well blended.
5. Cut each crispy chicken skin in 2 pieces.
6. Place 1 tablespoon Alfredo cheese mix on each chicken crisp and serve immediately.

PER 1 FAT BOMB Calories: 71 | Fat: 4g | Protein: 8g | Sodium: 65mg | Fiber: 0g | Carbohydrates: 1g | Sugar: 0g

Chicken Skin Crisps Satay DF

If you like Thai food, this fat-bomb recipe will absolutely delight you!

Prep Time: 5 minutes • Cook Time: 20 minutes

MAKES 6 FAT BOMBS

Skin from 3 chicken thighs

2 tablespoons chunky peanut butter

1 tablespoon coconut cream

1 teaspoon coconut oil

1 teaspoon seeded and minced fresh jalapeño pepper

¼ garlic clove, minced

1 teaspoon coconut aminos

> **Precious Liquid Fat**
>
> When you cook the chicken skins you will end up with a pan full of chicken fat. You can drain that into a glass jar and save it for later. This fat can be stored in the refrigerator for a couple of months and it can be used in any recipe as a 100 percent dairy-free substitute for butter.

1. Preheat oven to 350°F. On a cookie sheet, lay out skins as flat as possible.
2. Bake 12–15 minutes until skins turn light brown and crispy being careful not to burn them.
3. Remove skins from cookie sheet and place on a paper towel to cool.
4. In a small food processor, add peanut butter, coconut cream, coconut oil, jalapeño, garlic, and coconut aminos.
5. Mix about 30 seconds until well blended.
6. Cut each crispy chicken skin in 2 pieces.
7. Place 1 tablespoon peanut sauce on each chicken crisp and serve immediately. If sauce is too runny, refrigerate 2 hours before using.

PER 1 FAT BOMB Calories: 91 | Fat: 5g | Protein: 8g | Sodium: 105mg | Fiber: 0g | Carbohydrates: 3g | Sugar: 2g

Chicken Skin Crisps with Aioli Egg Salad DF

The rich, garlicky flavor of this fat bomb will transport you straight to the French Riviera.

Prep Time: 5 minutes • Cook Time: 20 minutes

MAKES 6 FAT BOMBS

Skin from 3 chicken thighs

1 large hard-boiled egg, peeled and chopped

1 large hard-boiled egg yolk, chopped

1 tablespoon mayonnaise

¼ garlic clove, minced

1 tablespoon finely chopped fresh parsley

½ teaspoon sea salt

> **The Power of Parsley**
> Parsley isn't just a garnish. The herb is rich in vitamin C and vitamin A, so it helps keep your immune system, bones, and nervous system strong. Parsley also helps flush out excess water from the body and keeps your kidneys healthy.

1. Preheat oven to 350°F. On a cookie sheet, lay out skins as flat as possible.
2. Bake 12–15 minutes until skins turn light brown and crispy being careful not to burn them.
3. Remove skins from cookie sheet and place on a paper towel to cool.
4. In a small bowl, add egg, egg yolk, mayonnaise, garlic, parsley, and sea salt.
5. Mix with a fork until well blended.
6. Cut each crispy chicken skin in 2 pieces.
7. Place 1 tablespoon egg salad mix on each chicken crisp and serve immediately.

PER 1 FAT BOMB Calories: 79 | Fat: 5g | Protein: 8g | Sodium: 252mg | Fiber: 0g | Carbohydrates: 0g | Sugar: 0g

Chicken Skin Crisps with Avocado and Cilantro DF

This tangy, salty, and crunchy treat will become one of your favorites! A true match made in heaven.

Prep Time: 5 minutes • Cook Time: 20 minutes

MAKES 6 FAT BOMBS

Skin from 3 chicken thighs
3 ounces (½ medium) avocado pulp
1 tablespoon finely chopped fresh cilantro
½ tablespoon melted chicken fat
½ tablespoon fresh lemon juice
½ tablespoon sea salt

1. Preheat oven to 350°F. On a cookie sheet, lay out skins as flat as possible.
2. Bake 12–15 minutes until skins turn light brown and crispy being careful not to burn them.
3. Remove skins from cookie sheet and place on a paper towel to cool.
4. Drain and reserve ½ tablespoon chicken fat from cookie sheet.
5. In a small bowl, combine avocado, cilantro, chicken fat, lemon juice, and sea salt.
6. Mix with a fork until well blended.
7. Cut each crispy chicken skin in 2 pieces.
8. Place 1 tablespoon avocado mix on each chicken crisp and serve immediately.

PER 1 FAT BOMB Calories: 78 | Fat: 5g | Protein: 7g | Sodium: 620mg | Fiber: 1g | Carbohydrates: 2g | Sugar: 0g

Chicken Skin Crisps with Spicy Avocado Cream

Sometimes a bit of spice is a great complement to the creaminess of an ingredient. That makes for a well-balanced recipe.

Prep Time: 5 minutes • Cook Time: 20 minutes

MAKES 6 FAT BOMBS

Skin from 3 chicken thighs
1½ ounces (¼ medium) avocado pulp
1½ ounces sour cream
½ fresh jalapeño pepper, seeded and finely chopped
½ teaspoon sea salt

1. Preheat oven to 350°F. On a cookie sheet lay, out skins as flat as possible.
2. Bake 12–15 minutes until skins turn light brown and crispy being careful not to burn them.
3. Remove skins from cookie sheet and place on a paper towel to cool.
4. In a small bowl, combine avocado pulp, sour cream, jalapeño, and sea salt.
5. Mix with a fork until well blended.
6. Cut each crispy chicken skin in 2 pieces.
7. Place 1 tablespoon avocado mix on each chicken crisp and serve immediately.

PER 1 FAT BOMB Calories: 66 | Fat: 4g | Protein: 7g | Sodium: 232mg | Fiber: 1g | Carbohydrates: 1g | Sugar: 0g

CHAPTER 6

Rollups

Smoked Salmon and Crème Fraîche Rollups

If you love a bagel and lox for breakfast or Sunday brunch, try this fat-bomb recipe instead. It will be just as satisfying and more rewarding as it helps you stay on track with the ketogenic way of eating.

Prep Time: 5 minutes • Cook Time: 0 minutes

MAKES 3 FAT BOMBS

3 ounces crème fraîche

⅛ teaspoon fresh lemon zest

3 slices smoked salmon (lox), about
   1 ounce each

> **Crème Fraîche**
> Crème fraîche is the French version of sour cream. Just like sour cream, it is a cultured cream, but it has lower acidity and higher fat content, which makes it the perfect ingredient for fat bombs!

1. In a small bowl, mix crème fraîche and lemon zest.
2. Spread ⅓ mixture on top of each salmon slice.
3. Roll slices into individual rolls and secure with a toothpick.
4. Serve immediately.

PER 1 FAT BOMB Calories: 87 | Fat: 7g | Protein: 6g |
Sodium: 245mg | Fiber: 0g | Carbohydrates: 8g | Sugar: 1g

Mediterranean Rollups DF

Olives and sun-dried tomatoes are the flavors of the Mediterranean Sea. From Italy to Greece, the tastes of hot summer days include ripe tomatoes and fresh olive oil, and the scent of beautiful olive groves. This recipe will take you there!

Prep Time: 7 minutes • Cook Time: 3 minutes

MAKES 2 FAT BOMBS

1 large egg
1 tablespoon extra-virgin olive oil
⅛ teaspoon sea salt
6 large kalamata olives, pitted
1 ounce sun-dried tomatoes in oil
⅛ teaspoon red chili flakes
⅛ teaspoon parsley flakes

1. In a small bowl, combine egg, olive oil, and salt and whisk until foamy.
2. Heat a small nonstick skillet over high heat and pour in egg mixture, spreading evenly so it forms a thin, even layer.
3. Once the first side is cooked, about 1 minute, flip frittata with the aid of a plate or a lid. Cook until golden on bottom, about 2 more minutes.
4. Remove frittata to a plate.
5. In a small food processor, mix olives, tomatoes, chili flakes, and parsley until well chopped and blended, about 30 seconds.
6. Spread olive paste on top of frittata in an even layer.
7. Roll frittata into a tight roll, cut into 2 pieces, and serve immediately.

PER 1 FAT BOMB Calories: 153 | Fat: 10g | Protein: 5g | Sodium: 478mg | Fiber: 2g | Carbohydrates: 14g | Sugar: 5g

Quattro Formaggi Rollups

Have you ever had quattro formaggi pizza? Can anyone resist this delicious blend of melted cheese? The kids will love it too.

Prep Time: 5 minutes • Cook Time: 5 minutes

MAKES 2 FAT BOMBS

1 large egg
1 tablespoon grated Parmesan
1 tablespoon crumbled blue cheese
1 teaspoon butter
1 tablespoon mascarpone
1 ounce thinly sliced Brie

1. In a small bowl, whisk egg, Parmesan, and blue cheese until foamy.
2. Heat a small nonstick skillet over high heat and melt butter.
3. Pour in egg mixture, spreading evenly so it forms a thin, even layer.
4. Once the first side is cooked, about 1 minute, flip frittata with the aid of a plate or a lid.
5. Spread mascarpone on top of frittata, then place Brie slices in the middle and cover with a lid.
6. Cook until golden on bottom, about 2 more minutes.
7. Remove frittata to a plate.
8. Roll frittata into a tight roll, cut into 2 pieces, and serve immediately while hot.

PER 1 FAT BOMB Calories: 152 | Fat: 13g | Protein: 9g | Sodium: 253mg | Fiber: 0g | Carbohydrates: 1g | Sugar: 1g

Salami and Olive Rollups

This recipe features more flavors of Italy . . . who doesn't love Italian food?

Prep Time: 5 minutes • Cook Time: 0 minutes

MAKES 3 FAT BOMBS

12 large kalamata olives, pitted

3 ounces cream cheese

3 (1-ounce) slices Italian salami

1. In a small food processor, mix olives and cream cheese until they form a coarse dough, about 10 seconds.
2. Form cheese mixture into 3 balls with the aid of a spoon.
3. Place each ball on a slice of salami, then roll salami around it and secure with a toothpick.
4. Serve immediately or refrigerate up to 3 days.

PER 1 FAT BOMB Calories: 233 | Fat: 20g | Protein: 8g | Sodium: 621mg | Fiber: 0g | Carbohydrates: 6g | Sugar: 1g

Smoked Salmon and Avocado Rollups DF

Super-quick and easy dairy-free fat bombs, these rollups make a great party food or an easy appetizer.

Prep Time: 5 minutes • Cook Time: 0 minutes

MAKES 3 FAT BOMBS

3 ounces (½ medium) avocado pulp

1 teaspoon fresh lemon juice

⅛ teaspoon sea salt

3 slices smoked salmon (lox), about 1 ounce each

1. In a small bowl, combine avocado, lemon juice, and salt; mash with a fork.
2. Spread ⅓ avocado mixture evenly on top of each salmon slice. Roll slices into individual rolls and secure with a toothpick.
3. Serve immediately.

PER 1 FAT BOMB Calories: 78 | Fat: 5g | Protein: 6g | Sodium: 320mg | Fiber: 2g | Carbohydrates: 2g | Sugar: 0g

CHAPTER 7

Baked Avocado

Creamy Rosemary and Prosciutto Baked Avocado

Have you ever tried the combination of rosemary and prosciutto? It's a perfect blend of savory flavors that will delight your taste buds and stimulate digestion.

Prep Time: 10 minutes • Cook Time: 20 minutes

MAKES 2 FAT BOMBS

1 medium avocado, halved and pitted, skin on
1 ounce cream cheese
1 tablespoon finely chopped fresh rosemary
1 ounce cooked prosciutto, crumbled

1. Preheat oven to 350°F.
2. Place avocado halves hole-side up in a shallow ramekin or ovenproof dish just large enough to hold them.
3. In a small bowl, mix cream cheese with rosemary and prosciutto.
4. Place ½ mixture into each avocado cavity.
5. Bake 20 minutes. Serve hot.

PER 1 FAT BOMB Calories: 226 | Fat: 20g | Protein: 5g | Sodium: 178mg | Fiber: 7g | Carbohydrates: 10g | Sugar: 1g

Baked Avocado with Blue Cheese

This is one of the easiest baked avocado recipes, but it is probably one of the most flavorful ones.

Prep Time: 10 minutes • Cook Time: 20 minutes

MAKES 2 FAT BOMBS
1 medium avocado, halved and pitted, skin on
2 ounces crumbled blue cheese
1 tablespoon butter, softened

1. Preheat oven to 350°F.
2. Place avocado halves hole-side up in a shallow ramekin or ovenproof dish just large enough to hold them.
3. In a small bowl, mix blue cheese and butter.
4. Place ½ mixture into each avocado cavity.
5. Bake 20 minutes. Serve hot.

PER 1 FAT BOMB Calories: 310 | Fat: 28g | Protein: 8g | Sodium: 398mg | Fiber: 7g | Carbohydrates: 9g | Sugar: 1g

Baked Avocado with Egg and Brie

A classic baked avocado and egg with a French twist!

Prep Time: 10 minutes • Cook Time: 20 minutes

MAKES 2 FAT BOMBS

1 medium avocado, halved and pitted, skin on

2 large egg yolks

1 ounce coarsely chopped Brie

¼ teaspoon freshly ground black pepper

1. Preheat oven to 350°F.
2. Place avocado halves hole-side up in a shallow ramekin or ovenproof dish just large enough to hold them.
3. Place 1 egg yolk into each avocado cavity. Divide Brie in half and place gently on top of egg yolks without breaking them. Season with pepper.
4. Bake 20 minutes. Serve hot.

PER 1 FAT BOMB Calories: 262 | Fat: 23g | Protein: 8g | Sodium: 103mg | Fiber: 7g | Carbohydrates: 9g | Sugar: 1g

Baked Avocado with Sriracha and Brie

This baked avocado features melted cheese, hot and creamy, with a bit of spice and garlic to create a complex harmony of flavors.

Prep Time: 10 minutes • Cook Time: 20 minutes

MAKES 2 FAT BOMBS

1 medium avocado, halved and pitted, skin on

1 ounce coarsely chopped Brie

½ teaspoon sriracha sauce

1. Preheat oven to 350°F.
2. Place avocado halves hole-side up in a shallow ramekin or ovenproof dish just large enough to hold them.
3. Mix Brie with sriracha sauce so it is evenly coated.
4. Divide Brie in half and place into each avocado cavity.
5. Bake 20 minutes. Serve hot.

PER 1 FAT BOMB Calories: 208 | Fat: 19g | Protein: 5g | Sodium: 101mg | Fiber: 7g | Carbohydrates: 9g | Sugar: 1g

Baked Egg Avocado DF

This super-easy recipe can become a quick go-to for breakfast or a snack.

Prep Time: 10 minutes • Cook Time: 20 minutes

MAKES 2 FAT BOMBS

1 medium avocado, halved and pitted, skin on

2 large egg yolks

2 teaspoons mayonnaise

¼ teaspoon freshly ground black pepper

> **Variation on Baked Egg Avocado**
> You can make an easy variation here by swirling together the mayonnaise and the egg yolk in the cavity of the avocado. The yolk will then cook more evenly throughout.

1. Preheat oven to 350°F.
2. Place avocado halves hole-side up in a shallow ramekin or ovenproof dish just large enough to hold them.
3. Place 1 egg yolk into each avocado cavity.
4. In a small bowl, mix mayonnaise and black pepper and then divide between avocado halves, placing gently on top of each egg yolk without breaking it.
5. Bake 20 minutes. Serve hot.

PER 1 FAT BOMB Calories: 248 | Fat: 23g | Protein: 5g | Sodium: 41mg | Fiber: 7g | Carbohydrates: 9g | Sugar: 8g

Crab Dynamite Baked Avocado DF

Are you familiar with the Japanese dish Dynamite? It consists of different kinds of fish and scallops mixed with mayonnaise, and then is cooked under the broiler. This is an easy home version using avocado and crabmeat as a fat bomb!

Prep Time: 10 minutes • Cook Time: 20 minutes

MAKES 2 FAT BOMBS

1 medium avocado, halved and pitted, skin on

1½ ounces real crabmeat, drained from juices

2 teaspoons mayonnaise

1 teaspoon coconut aminos or tamari

¼ teaspoon freshly ground black pepper

Soy-Free Coconut Aminos

Coconut aminos is a great substitution for soy sauce for people who prefer not using any soy products. Coconut aminos can be purchased through many major retailers online and in stores.

1. Preheat oven to 350°F.
2. Place avocado halves hole-side up in a shallow ramekin or ovenproof dish just large enough to hold them.
3. Mix crabmeat, mayonnaise, coconut aminos, and pepper in a small bowl, then divide and scoop into each avocado cavity.
4. Bake 20 minutes. Serve hot.

PER 1 FAT BOMB Calories: 217 | Fat: 19g | Protein: 7g | Sodium: 253mg | Fiber: 7g | Carbohydrates: 9g | Sugar: 1g

Savory-Sweet Baked Avocado with Pecans and Coconut DF

This is another recipe that mixes savory and sweet. This one has a subtle sweetness but no added sugar.

Prep Time: 10 minutes • Cook Time: 20 minutes

MAKES 2 FAT BOMBS

1 medium avocado, halved and pitted, skin on

2 tablespoons grated unsweetened coconut

2 tablespoons coconut oil

6 pecan halves

Taste Enhancer!
You will find that once you reduce the amount of sugar you consume, your taste buds will reset. You'll start enjoying much wider nuances of flavor!

1. Preheat oven to 350°F.
2. Place avocado halves hole-side up in a shallow ramekin or ovenproof dish just large enough to hold them.
3. Mix grated coconut with coconut oil in a small bowl and scoop into each avocado cavity.
4. Place 3 pecans on top of each avocado half, gently nudging them in.
5. Bake 20 minutes. Serve hot or cold.

PER 1 FAT BOMB Calories: 328 | Fat: 33g | Protein: 3g | Sodium: 8mg | Fiber: 8g | Carbohydrates: 10g | Sugar: 1g

Smoked Salmon and Brie Baked Avocado

Smoked salmon and Brie are a classic combination. These avocados are great served cold, but are so much better when hot and melted!

Prep Time: 10 minutes • Cook Time: 20 minutes

MAKES 2 FAT BOMBS

1 medium avocado, halved and pitted, skin on
1½ ounces wild-caught smoked salmon, coarsely chopped
1 tablespoon plus 1 teaspoon Brie
¼ teaspoon freshly ground black pepper

1. Preheat oven to 350°F.
2. Place avocado halves hole-side up in a shallow ramekin or ovenproof dish just large enough to hold them.
3. Mix salmon, Brie, and pepper in a small bowl, then scoop ½ mixture into each avocado cavity.
4. Bake 20 minutes. Serve hot.

PER 1 FAT BOMB Calories: 221 | Fat: 19g | Protein: 8g | Sodium: 238mg | Fiber: 7g | Carbohydrates: 8g | Sugar: 1g

CHAPTER 8

Savory Panna Cotta

Goat Cheese and Herbs Panna Cotta

Herbed goat cheese is a very popular item in fancy cheese stores. Now you can replicate that fancy flavor with the right amount of good fat for your keto diet.

Prep Time: 6–12 hours • Cook Time: 10 minutes

MAKES 6 FAT BOMBS

1½ cups heavy whipping cream
¾ cup sour cream
6 ounces soft goat cheese
1 teaspoon Herbes de Provence
2 teaspoons powdered unflavored gelatin
1 teaspoon sea salt

1. In a small saucepan over medium heat, combine heavy cream, sour cream, goat cheese, and Herbes de Provence, stirring until cheese melts.
2. Whisk in gelatin and salt until completely incorporated.
3. Simmer on very low heat about 5 minutes, stirring constantly.
4. Pour mixture evenly into 6 small glasses or ramekins.
5. Refrigerate until set, at least 6 hours or overnight.
6. Serve in glass or invert over a small plate after dipping glass into hot water a few seconds.

PER 1 FAT BOMB Calories: 397 | Fat: 38g | Protein: 11g | Sodium: 537mg | Fiber: 0g | Carbohydrates: 3g | Sugar: 2g

Gorgonzola Panna Cotta

This is the kind of recipe you would eat at a dinner party or in a fancy restaurant. Isn't it wonderful that even the fanciest recipes can sometimes be as easy as they are delicious?

Prep Time: 6–12 hours • Cook Time: 5 minutes

MAKES 6 FAT BOMBS

12 ounces crumbled Gorgonzola or blue cheese

1½ cups heavy whipping cream

2 teaspoons powdered unflavored gelatin

12 pecan halves

How to Serve Panna Cotta

You can serve panna cotta in a small pretty glass or cup, so it can be eaten with a spoon as a mousse might be served. The other option is to use a mold or ramekin, so it can be inverted onto a plate. If you chose this option, right before serving, dip each ramekin three-quarters of the way in warm water to loosen the panna cotta, then invert onto a plate.

1. In a small saucepan over medium heat, melt Gorgonzola in heavy cream using a whisk to break clots, about 2 minutes.

2. Whisk in gelatin until completely incorporated.

3. Pour mixture evenly into 6 small glasses or ramekins.

4. Refrigerate until set, at least 6 hours or overnight.

5. Decorate each glass with 2 pecan halves and serve.

PER 1 FAT BOMB Calories: 435 | Fat: 41g | Protein: 14g | Sodium: 1,037mg | Fiber: 0g | Carbohydrates: 3g | Sugar: 0g

Porcini Mushroom Panna Cotta

This recipe will make a great impression on the guests of a dinner party . . . and they will never know you are just serving a fat bomb.

Prep Time: 6½–12 hours • Cook Time: 5 minutes

MAKES 6 FAT BOMBS

2 ounces dried porcini mushrooms

1 cup hot water

1 teaspoon powdered unflavored gelatin

1 tablespoon butter

1 cup heavy cream

1 tablespoon coconut aminos

3 tablespoons grated Parmesan

Skip the Soy
Coconut aminos sauce is a soy-free seasoning alternative made from the sap of coconut blossoms that you can use in place of soy sauce in any of your recipes. There is absolutely no coconut flavor—it tastes just like soy sauce—but unlike soy sauce, which is highly processed and most likely contains GMOs, coconut aminos is GMO-free and contains seventeen amino acids, vitamins, and minerals.

1. Soak porcini mushrooms in hot water about 30 minutes to rehydrate.
2. Drain mushrooms, reserving the soaking water. Squeeze out excess water from mushrooms, then chop finely.
3. Place 3 tablespoons soaking water in a glass. Sprinkle gelatin in soaking water and let stand about 5 minutes.
4. In a small nonstick skillet over high heat, melt butter, then add mushrooms and sauté about 3 minutes, stirring.
5. Add soaking water with gelatin, cream, coconut aminos, and Parmesan; stir and bring to a boil, about 1 minute.
6. Remove from heat.
7. Pour mixture evenly into 6 small glasses or ramekins.
8. Refrigerate until set, at least 6 hours or overnight.
9. Serve in glass or invert over a small plate after dipping glass into hot water a few seconds.

PER 1 FAT BOMB Calories: 188 | Fat: 19g | Protein: 4g | Sodium: 274mg | Fiber: 0g | Carbohydrates: 2g | Sugar: 0g

Sour Cream and Rosemary Panna Cotta

This recipe features easy everyday ingredients with an unusual flavor combination. Impress your taste buds.

Prep Time: 6–12 hours • Cook Time: 7 minutes

MAKES 6 FAT BOMBS

1½ cups heavy whipping cream

1½ cups sour cream

2 medium sprigs fresh rosemary, plus extra leaves for garnish

2 teaspoons powdered unflavored gelatin

1 teaspoon sea salt

Infusing Rosemary Flavor Into Your Cream

As you are simmering the cream with the rosemary, smash the rosemary sprigs with the tip of the whisk gently enough to release some of the oils but without breaking off pieces.

1. In a small saucepan over medium heat, combine heavy cream, sour cream, and rosemary sprigs. Stir until melted together.
2. Whisk in gelatin and salt until completely incorporated.
3. Simmer on very low heat about 5 minutes, stirring constantly.
4. With a fork, remove rosemary sprigs from cream.
5. Pour mixture evenly into 6 small glasses or ramekins.
6. Refrigerate until set, at least 6 hours or overnight.
7. Decorate each glass with a few rosemary leaves and serve.

PER 1 FAT BOMB Calories: 332 | Fat: 34g | Protein: 3g | Sodium: 466mg | Fiber: 1g | Carbohydrates: 5g | Sugar: 2g

Sage Panna Cotta

The delicate flavor of sage superbly complements the smoothness of cream.

Prep Time: 6–12 hours • Cook Time: 20 minutes

MAKES 6 FAT BOMBS

8–10 fresh sage leaves

1½ cups heavy cream

12 ounces cream cheese

1 tablespoon powdered unflavored gelatin

½ tablespoon sea salt

> **Be Choosy with Dairy**
>
> Heavy cream, cheese, and butter are staples on a ketogenic diet, but some dairy products are filled with hormones. Choose grass-fed butter and organic heavy cream whenever possible.

1. In a small saucepan over low heat, immerse sage in cream and simmer 5 minutes. Then let sit an additional 5–10 minutes to infuse.
2. Remove sage from cream and reheat cream over very low heat.
3. Add cream cheese and whisk until completely melted.
4. Whisk in gelatin and salt until incorporated.
5. Pour mixture evenly into 6 small glasses or ramekins.
6. Refrigerate until set, at least 6 hours or overnight.
7. Serve in glass or invert over a small plate after dipping glass into hot water a few seconds.

PER 1 FAT BOMB Calories: 402 | Fat: 41g | Protein: 6g | Sodium: 794mg | Fiber: 0g | Carbohydrates: 4g | Sugar: 2g

Turmeric-Infused Panna Cotta DF

Turmeric used to be considered an exotic spice, but it is now widely available in any supermarket, even the fresh root version. Try this pungent condiment, and the earthy but distinct flavor will surely win you over.

Prep Time: 6–12 hours • Cook Time: 8 minutes

MAKES 6 FAT BOMBS

1½ cups coconut milk, refrigerated and cream separated from the water

1½ cups homemade beef stock

1½ tablespoons powdered unflavored gelatin

1 tablespoon turmeric

½ tablespoon sea salt

The Benefits of Turmeric

The main active ingredient in turmeric, called curcumin (not to be confused with the common spice, cumin), is recognized as being a powerful anti-inflammatory. Even a small serving in a dish can assist your body's ability to digest fats and reduce bloating. It's also used medicinally to provide relief to sufferers of joint pain and swelling.

1. In a small saucepan over medium heat, heat coconut cream and beef stock.
2. Whisk in gelatin until completely incorporated.
3. Add turmeric and salt and simmer 5 minutes.
4. Pour mixture evenly into 6 small glasses or ramekins.
5. Refrigerate until set, at least 6 hours or overnight.
6. Serve in glass or invert over a small plate after dipping glass into hot water a few seconds.

PER 1 FAT BOMB Calories: 130 | Fat: 12g | Protein: 4g | Sodium: 719mg | Fiber: 0g | Carbohydrates: 3g | Sugar: 0g

CHAPTER 9

Prosciutto, Bacon, and Endive Cups

Baked Brie and Pecan Prosciutto Cup

Be adventurous and try mixing sweet and savory flavors to make unusual but tasty combinations. You may be surprised by the delicious results.

Prep Time: 20 minutes • Cook Time: 12 minutes

MAKES 1 FAT BOMB

1 slice prosciutto (about ½ ounce)
1 ounce Brie, diced with white skin on
6 pecan halves (about ⅓ ounce)
⅛ teaspoon freshly ground black pepper

> **Melting and Delicious**
>
> You can make a batch of these fat bombs; just multiply the amount of ingredients by the number of servings you'd like to create. However, they do taste better when warm and the Brie is melting, so it's best to make a single recipe at a time for yourself.

1. Preheat oven to 350°F. Use a muffin tin with holes about 2½" wide and 1½" deep.
2. Fold prosciutto slice in half so it becomes almost square.
3. Place it in muffin tin hole to line it completely.
4. Place Brie in prosciutto-lined cup.
5. Stick pecan halves in amongst Brie.
6. Bake about 12 minutes until Brie is melted and prosciutto is cooked.
7. Let cool 10 minutes before removing from muffin pan.

PER 1 FAT BOMB Calories: 182 | Fat: 15g | Protein: 12g | Sodium: 462mg | Fiber: 1g | Carbohydrates: 2g | Sugar: 1g

Cheesy Muffin Prosciutto Cup

Salty prosciutto, creamy melted cheeses, and a nourishing egg—sounds like a perfect combination.

Prep Time: 20 minutes • Cook Time: 12 minutes

MAKES 1 FAT BOMB

1 slice prosciutto (about ½ ounce)
1 medium egg yolk
½ ounce diced Brie
⅓ ounce diced mozzarella
½ ounce grated Parmesan

1. Preheat oven to 350°F. Use a muffin tin with holes about 2½" wide and 1½" deep.
2. Fold prosciutto slice in half so it becomes almost square.
3. Place it in muffin tin hole to line it completely.
4. Place egg yolk into prosciutto cup.
5. Add cheeses on top of egg yolk gently without breaking it.
6. Bake about 12 minutes until yolk is cooked and warm but still runny.
7. Let cool 10 minutes before removing from muffin pan.

PER 1 FAT BOMB Calories: 218 | Fat: 15g | Protein: 18g | Sodium: 655mg | Fiber: 0g | Carbohydrates: 2g | Sugar: 0g

Kalamata Olive and Brie Prosciutto Cup

Don't you love the flavor of olives? Not only do they have a very rich flavor, they also provide great fats and very little carbs—perfect for a fat bomb!

Prep Time: 20 minutes • Cook Time: 12 minutes

MAKES 1 FAT BOMB

1 slice prosciutto
1 medium egg
1 ounce diced Brie
4 large kalamata olives, pitted and chopped
¼ teaspoon Herbes de Provence

> **Herbes de Provence**
> Herbes de Provence is a mixture of dried herbs typical of the Provence region of southeast France. This mixture usually contains savory, marjoram, rosemary, thyme, oregano, and other herbs. In the North American market, lavender leaves are also typically included.

1. Preheat oven to 350°F. Use a muffin tin with holes about 2½" wide and 1½" deep.
2. Fold prosciutto slice in half so it becomes almost square.
3. Place it in a muffin tin hole to line it completely.
4. Break egg into prosciutto cup.
5. Gently place Brie and olives on top of egg. Sprinkle with Herbes de Provence.
6. Bake about 12 minutes until egg white is cooked and yolk is still runny but warm.
7. Let cool 10 minutes before removing from muffin pan.

PER 1 FAT BOMB Calories: 241 | Fat: 13g | Protein: 17g | Sodium: 529mg | Fiber: 1g | Carbohydrates: 15g | Sugar: 0g

Egg and Mascarpone Prosciutto Cup

This fat bomb can become a whole breakfast! Great taste, nutrition, and the right macronutrient ratios to start your day.

Prep Time: 20 minutes • Cook Time: 12 minutes

MAKES 1 FAT BOMB

1 slice prosciutto
1 medium egg
1 tablespoon mascarpone

1. Preheat oven to 350°F. Use a muffin tin with holes about 2½" wide and 1½" deep.
2. Fold prosciutto slice in half so it becomes almost square.
3. Place it in a muffin tin hole to line it completely.
4. Break egg into prosciutto cup.
5. Gently place mascarpone on top of egg.
6. Bake about 12 minutes until egg white is cooked and yolk is still runny but warm.
7. Let cool 10 minutes before removing from muffin pan.

PER 1 FAT BOMB Calories: 141 | Fat: 10g | Protein: 11g |
Sodium: 394mg | Fiber: 0g | Carbohydrates: 1g | Sugar: 1g

Olive Dynamite Prosciutto Cup DF

Have you ever tried baking mayonnaise, like in the Japanese Dynamite dish? It actually pairs well with more than just fish!

Prep Time: 20 minutes • Cook Time: 12 minutes

MAKES 1 FAT BOMB

1 slice prosciutto
1 medium egg yolk
1 tablespoon olive oil mayonnaise
4 large kalamata olives, pitted and chopped
¼ teaspoon Herbes de Provence

1. Preheat oven to 350°F. Use a muffin tin with holes about 2½" wide and 1½" deep.
2. Fold prosciutto slice in half so it becomes almost square.
3. Place it in a muffin tin hole to line it completely.
4. Break egg yolk into prosciutto cup.
5. Gently place mayonnaise and olives on top of egg. Sprinkle with Herbes de Provence.
6. Bake about 12 minutes until egg yolk is still runny but warm.
7. Let cool 10 minutes before removing from muffin pan.

PER 1 FAT BOMB Calories: 209 | Fat: 16g | Protein: 8g | Sodium: 376mg | Fiber: 1g | Carbohydrates: 8g | Sugar: 0g

Hot Mess Prosciutto Cup

Hot and dripping with melted cheese, how do you like this version of a hot mess? Couldn't you eat this every day?

Prep Time: 20 minutes • Cook Time: 12 minutes

MAKES 1 FAT BOMB

1 slice prosciutto
1 medium egg yolk
½ ounce diced Brie
½ ounce grated Parmesan
½ teaspoon sriracha sauce

1. Preheat oven to 350°F. Use a muffin tin with holes about 2½" wide and 1½" deep.
2. Fold prosciutto slice in half so it becomes almost square.
3. Place it in a muffin tin hole to line it completely.
4. Place egg yolk into prosciutto cup.
5. Add cheeses on top of egg gently without breaking it.
6. Add sriracha sauce on top of everything.
7. Bake about 12 minutes until yolk is cooked and warm but still runny.
8. Let cool 10 minutes before removing from muffin pan.

PER 1 FAT BOMB Calories: 190 | Fat: 13g | Protein: 16g |
Sodium: 659mg | Fiber: 0g | Carbohydrates: 1g | Sugar: 0g

Egg and Avocado Bacon Cups DF

Bacon cups make an excellent replacement for bread or crackers for those following a low-carb, high-fat diet. This combination successfully uses bacon in place of bread to serve up a delicious avocado egg salad.

Prep Time: 30 minutes • Cook Time: 12–15 minutes

MAKES 6 FAT BOMBS

12 slices regular-cut bacon, 6 cut in half

1 medium avocado, pitted, peeled, and diced

4 large hard-boiled eggs, peeled and diced

½ teaspoon salt

⅛ teaspoon freshly ground black pepper

> **What Is an Avocado Anyway?**
> While most people know that avocado is full of healthy fats, they would be hard pressed to tell you the avocado is actually a fruit. To be more specific, the avocado is a berry. Surprised?

1. Preheat oven to 400°F.
2. In a standard-sized muffin tin, place half-strips bacon in an *X* shape in the bottom of 6 cups. Line those same cups with 1 full slice bacon along the inside of the cup vertically.
3. Place a cookie sheet underneath muffin tin and bake cups 12–15 minutes until slightly browned and crisp.
4. While cups are baking, mash avocado, eggs, salt, and pepper in a medium mixing bowl. Cover and set in refrigerator to chill.
5. After bacon cups have cooled, fill with egg mixture and serve.

PER 1 FAT BOMB Calories: 309 | Fat: 29g | Protein: 10g | Sodium: 623mg | Fiber: 2g | Carbohydrates: 3g | Sugar: 0g

Egg, Sausage, and Chorizo Bacon Cups DF

These classic flavors combine to make a portable, low-carbohydrate breakfast bowl. This bowl is a truly filling meal for any pork lover on the run.

Prep Time: 10 minutes • Cook Time: 20–25 minutes

MAKES 6 FAT BOMBS
12 slices regular-cut bacon, 6 cut in half
4 large eggs
½ teaspoon salt
2 tablespoons freshly chopped cilantro
4 ounces raw breakfast sausage
2 ounces raw chorizo
¼ small yellow onion, peeled and diced

1. Preheat oven to 400°F.
2. In a standard-sized muffin tin, place half-strips bacon in an *X* shape in the bottom of 6 cups. Line those same cups with a full slice of bacon along the inside of the cup vertically.
3. Place a cookie sheet underneath muffin tin and bake cups 8–10 minutes until they're a little pliable.
4. While cups are precooking, scramble eggs with salt and cilantro in a medium bowl. Set aside.
5. Combine breakfast sausage, chorizo, and onions in small mixing bowl.
6. Take cups out of oven and divide chorizo and sausage mixture equally between cups.
7. Pour egg mixture over sausage mixture and return cups to oven.
8. Bake cups 12–15 minutes more until eggs set. Serve warm.

PER 1 FAT BOMB Calories: 356 | Fat: 32g | Protein: 15g | Sodium: 855mg | Fiber: 0g | Carbohydrates: 1g | Sugar: 0g

Egg, Sour Cream, and Chive Bacon Cups

Sour cream is an excellent way to add extra fat to your fat bombs, and to make scrambled eggs taste even creamier. Chives enhance the flavor to make this cup even better than a potato chip with a similar name.

Prep Time: 10 minutes • Cook Time: 16–20 minutes

MAKES 6 FAT BOMBS

12 slices regular-cut bacon, 6 cut in half
4 large eggs
½ teaspoon salt
¼ teaspoon freshly ground black pepper
2 tablespoons diced chives
2 tablespoons sour cream

1. Preheat oven to 400°F.
2. In a standard-sized muffin tin, place half-strips in an *X* shape in the bottom of 6 cups. Line those same cups with 1 full slice bacon along the inside of the cup vertically.
3. Place a cookie sheet underneath muffin tin and bake cups 8–10 minutes until they're a little pliable.
4. While cups are precooking, scramble eggs with remaining ingredients in a medium bowl. Set aside.
5. Take cups out of oven and divide egg mixture equally between cups.
6. Bake cups 8–10 minutes more until eggs set. Serve warm.

PER 1 FAT BOMB Calories: 265 | Fat: 25g | Protein: 10g | Sodium: 625mg | Fiber: 0g | Carbohydrates: 1g | Sugar: 0g

Smoked Salmon Mousse Bacon Cups

The salty crunch of bacon surrounding a luscious, creamy salmon mousse is the definition of decadence. Intensifying the flavor with fresh herbs only adds to the gourmet taste of this fantastic finger food.

Prep Time: 15 minutes • Cook Time: 12–15 minutes

MAKES 6 FAT BOMBS

12 slices regular-cut bacon, 6 cut in half
6 ounces smoked salmon
4 ounces cream cheese, softened
1 tablespoon heavy whipping cream
⅛ teaspoon freshly ground black pepper
1 teaspoon fresh dill, plus 6 sprigs for garnish

A Little Lox Lesson

While lox is generally a salted, not smoked, salmon, it is a popular way to serve salmon with cream cheese. Salted salmon, also known as lox, became a popular staple with Jewish immigrants in the late 1800s in America, but the mystery of when it was first combined with cream cheese, capers, red onion, and a bagel still remains.

1. Preheat oven to 400°F.
2. In a standard-sized muffin tin, place half-strips bacon in an *X* shape in the bottom of 6 cups. Line those same cups with 1 full slice bacon along the inside of the cup vertically.
3. Place a cookie sheet underneath muffin tin and bake cups 12–15 minutes until slightly browned and crisp.
4. While cups are baking, combine remaining ingredients in a food processor and pulse until smooth. Cover and set in refrigerator to chill.
5. After bacon cups have cooled, fill with mousse mixture and serve with a fresh sprig of dill on top.

PER 1 FAT BOMB Calories: 312 | Fat: 29g | Protein: 12g | Sodium: 658mg | Fiber: 0g | Carbohydrates: 1g | Sugar: 1g

Nutty Bacon Baskets

Another delicious combination of savory flavors and sweet nuts. These bacon cups will delight your taste buds.

Prep Time: 15 minutes • Cook Time: 12–15 minutes

MAKES 6 FAT BOMBS

12 slices regular-cut bacon, 6 cut in half

1 tablespoon butter

½ cup pecans

½ cup macadamia nuts

¼ teaspoon granulated garlic

⅛ teaspoon freshly ground black pepper

4 slices cooked bacon, chopped into bits

> ### Crunchy Comfort Food Combo
> While it may not seem to be a likely pair, salty bacon and nuts make an excellent duo. The crispiness of the bacon and the crunchy, subtle sweetness of the nuts provide a perfect balance of flavors. One thing is certain about these bacon cups: They will be hard to keep away from the men in your life.

1. Preheat oven to 400°F.

2. In a standard-sized muffin tin, place half-strips bacon in an *X* shape in the bottom of 6 cups. Line those same cups with 1 full slice bacon along the inside of the cup vertically.

3. Place a cookie sheet underneath muffin tin and bake cups 12–15 minutes until slightly browned and crisp.

4. While cups are baking, melt butter over medium-low heat in a medium skillet. Add nuts, garlic, and pepper and cook 2–3 minutes. Remove from heat.

5. Once cooled, coarsely chop nut mixture and combine with bacon bits.

6. Divide nut mixture between cups and serve.

PER 1 FAT BOMB Calories: 437 | Fat: 44g | Protein: 9g | Sodium: 504mg | Fiber: 2g | Carbohydrates: 3g | Sugar: 1g

Crab and Avocado Endive Cups DF

Crab can be tasty in many different ways, not just in crab cakes.

Prep Time: 5 minutes • Cook Time: 0 minutes

MAKES 4 FAT BOMBS

1 ounce canned crabmeat, drained
1 ounce avocado pulp
1 teaspoon finely chopped cilantro
1 tablespoon chopped green onion
1 teaspoon fresh lime juice
1 tablespoon coconut oil
⅛ teaspoon sea salt
⅛ teaspoon freshly ground black pepper
4 Belgian endive leaves, washed and dried

1. In a small food processor, mix all ingredients except endive until well blended.
2. Scoop 1 tablespoon crab mix onto each endive cup.
3. Serve immediately.

PER 1 FAT BOMB Calories: 51 | Fat: 5g | Protein: 2g |
Sodium: 98mg | Fiber: 1g | Carbohydrates: 1g | Sugar: 0g

Creamy Tuna Endive Cups

A super-simple, super-quick recipe that can save your lunch in a moment.

Prep Time: 5 minutes • Cook Time: 0 minutes

MAKES 4 FAT BOMBS

1 ounce canned tuna in olive oil, drained

1 ounce cream cheese

4 Belgian endive leaves, washed and dried

2 tablespoons hemp hearts

1. In a small food processor, mix tuna and cream cheese until well blended.
2. Scoop 1 tablespoon tuna cream onto each endive cup.
3. Sprinkle ½ tablespoon hemp hearts over each endive cup. Serve immediately.

PER 1 FAT BOMB Calories: 46 | Fat: 3g | Protein: 3g | Sodium: 47mg | Fiber: 0g | Carbohydrates: 2g | Sugar: 0g

Curried Egg Salad Endive Cups DF

The delicate but complex flavor of the curry blends wonderfully with eggs, giving the egg salad a slightly unusual but successful twist.

Prep Time: 5 minutes • Cook Time: 0 minutes

MAKES 2 FAT BOMBS

1 large hard-boiled egg, peeled

1 teaspoon curry powder

1 tablespoon coconut oil

⅛ teaspoon sea salt

⅛ teaspoon freshly ground black pepper

2 Belgian endive leaves, washed and dried

1. In a small food processor, mix all ingredients except endive until well blended.
2. Scoop 1 tablespoon egg salad mix onto each endive cup.
3. Serve immediately.

PER 1 FAT BOMB Calories: 102 | Fat: 9g | Protein: 3g | Sodium: 183mg | Fiber: 1g | Carbohydrates: 1g | Sugar: 0g

Kitchen Sink Endive Cups DF

This recipe has a bit of every good fat and protein you can use in your kitchen on a daily basis.

Prep Time: 5 minutes • Cook Time: 0 minutes

MAKES 4 FAT BOMBS

1 large hard-boiled egg, peeled

1 ounce canned tuna in olive oil, drained

1 ounce avocado pulp

1 teaspoon fresh lime juice

1 tablespoon mayonnaise

⅛ teaspoon sea salt

⅛ teaspoon freshly ground black pepper

4 Belgian endive leaves, washed and dried

1. In a small food processor, mix all ingredients except endive until well blended.
2. Scoop 1 tablespoon tuna mix onto each endive cup.
3. Serve immediately.

PER 1 FAT BOMB Calories: 69 | Fat: 6g | Protein: 4g | Sodium: 136mg | Fiber: 1g | Carbohydrates: 1g | Sugar: 0g

Tuna and Olive Endive Cups DF

Another recipe inspired form the glorious country of Italy, with the best food in the world.

Prep Time: 5 minutes • Cook Time: 0 minutes

MAKES 4 FAT BOMBS

1 ounce canned tuna in olive oil, drained

6 large kalamata olives, pitted

½ tablespoon chopped green onion

1 teaspoon extra-virgin olive oil

4 Belgian endive leaves, washed and dried

1. In a small food processor mix tuna, olives, green onion, and olive oil until well blended.
2. Scoop 1 tablespoon tuna mix onto each endive cup.
3. Serve immediately.

PER 1 FAT BOMB Calories: 29 | Fat: 2g | Protein: 2g | Sodium: 25mg | Fiber: 0g | Carbohydrates: 1g | Sugar: 0g

CHAPTER 10

Baked Finger Foods

Chorizo-Stuffed Jalapeños

There is perhaps no better pairing than chorizo with spicy peppers baked into a delicious creamy mound of cheese. The addition of bacon is truly the icing on the cake.

Prep Time: 15 minutes • Cook Time: 15–22 minutes

MAKES 6 FAT BOMBS

1 tablespoon olive oil

¼ medium yellow onion, peeled and minced

6 ounces pork chorizo sausage

4 ounces cream cheese, softened to room temperature

3 medium jalapeño peppers, seeded and sliced in half

3 slices bacon, sliced in half horizontally

> **Why Do Americans Love Jalapeño Poppers?**
> Although their origin is a bit fuzzy, poppers were speculated to be an American spinoff of the Mexican classic chili rellenos. Nobody can seem to pinpoint who coined the term "poppers" and decided to batter dip, freeze, and commercialize them in the 1980s, but they have been a popular restaurant staple in California restaurants since at least the 1960s.

1. Preheat oven to 375°F.
2. Add olive oil to a medium skillet over medium heat and sweat onion 2 minutes. Add chorizo to pan and cook another 3–5 minutes. Drain mixture.
3. In mixing bowl, whip softened cream cheese with hand mixer until softened. Fold in sausage and onion mixture with a spatula.
4. Stuff each pepper half with sausage mixture.
5. Wrap 1 bacon slice around each stuffed pepper in a spiral motion, covering the cheese mixture underneath.
6. Bake 10–15 minutes or until bacon becomes crispy and cheese mixture underneath bubbles through and turns slightly brown. Serve warm.

PER 1 FAT BOMB Calories: 448 | Fat: 42g | Protein: 14g | Sodium: 665mg | Fiber: 0g | Carbohydrates: 3g | Sugar: 2g

Stuffed Baby Bella Mushroom Caps

Mushrooms make an excellent holder for meat-based fat bombs. These bombs use a hearty and earthy-tasting mushroom filled with the proper proportion of tangy cheese and savory sausage.

Prep Time: 10 minutes • Cook Time: 20 minutes

MAKES 8 FAT BOMBS

1 tablespoon olive oil
8 baby bella mushrooms, cleaned and stems removed
¼ teaspoon salt
4 ounces pork breakfast sausage, at room temperature
4 tablespoons chopped parsley
½ cup shredded Parmesan

1. Preheat oven to 350°F.
2. Rub olive oil on mushroom tops and sprinkle lightly with salt.
3. Mix sausage, parsley, and cheese in a small mixing bowl.
4. Stuff each mushroom cap until mixture forms a nice cap slightly above the mushroom ribbing.
5. Bake on a cookie sheet roughly 20 minutes until sausage becomes browned and cheese browns slightly. Serve warm.

PER 1 FAT BOMB Calories: 460 | Fat: 36g | Protein: 30g | Sodium: 1,554mg | Fiber: 1g | Carbohydrates: 4g | Sugar: 1g

Bacon-Wrapped Asparagus DF

This easy and elegant finger food makes a delicious appetizer that suits almost any diet. The crispiness of asparagus when prepared in this manner pairs so well with the crunchy, salty bacon. Even those who don't like this vegetable may have a change of heart when they try this recipe!

Prep Time: 5 minutes • Cook Time: 7–10 minutes

MAKES 4 FAT BOMBS

12 spears asparagus, rinsed with bottoms snapped off

1 tablespoon olive oil

⅛ teaspoon salt

⅛ teaspoon freshly ground black pepper

8 slices bacon

½ lemon, juiced

> **What's So Great about Asparagus Anyway?**
>
> With so many beneficial vitamins and nutrients, including vitamins A, K, C, and E, most would consider this a power-packed vegetable. Add to that the mineral chromium and antioxidant glutathione, and now it becomes a blood-sugar-reducing, detoxifying powerhouse.

1. Preheat oven to 375°F.
2. Thoroughly coat asparagus with olive oil and sprinkle with salt and pepper.
3. Bundle 3 spears asparagus together and wrap in a spiral fashion from top to bottom with 2 slices bacon.
4. Lay flat on cookie sheet and bake 7–10 minutes until bacon crisps and asparagus turns bright green.
5. Remove from oven and squeeze fresh lemon over spears. Serve warm.

PER 1 FAT BOMB Calories: 247 | Fat: 24g | Protein: 6g | Sodium: 452mg | Fiber: 1g | Carbohydrates: 2g | Sugar: 1g

Bacon Lovin' Onion Bites

This recipe will be a hit with the boys on game day or as a healthy appetizer for a gathering. But that doesn't mean you can't enjoy them on a daily basis!

Prep Time: 20 minutes • Cook Time: 25–30 minutes

MAKES 4 FAT BOMBS

1 large yellow onion

½ pound 80/20 ground chuck

¼ cup diced yellow onion

¼ cup diced mushrooms

2 tablespoons freshly chopped Italian parsley

¼ teaspoon salt

⅛ teaspoon cayenne pepper

1 large egg

½ teaspoon Worcestershire sauce

1 tablespoon coconut oil, melted

12 slices bacon

1 tablespoon butter, melted

1 teaspoon powdered stevia

1. Preheat oven to 350°F.
2. Cut off top and bottom of large onion. Peel skin. Cut in half vertically. Save 4 of the outside layers for a total of 8 halves.
3. In a large mixing bowl, mix meat with diced vegetables, parsley, salt, and cayenne.
4. In a small mixing bowl, whisk together egg, Worcestershire sauce, and coconut oil. Pour over meat mixture and knead together.
5. Form meat into 4 equal-sized balls and surround each ball with 2 onion halves. Wrap each ball with 3 pieces bacon and secure with toothpicks if needed to keep the balls together.
6. Place balls into a shallow baking tray.
7. In a small bowl or cup, mix melted butter and stevia and brush over bacon-wrapped onion balls.
8. Bake 25–30 minutes until bacon is crisped and browned. Serve warm.

PER 1 FAT BOMB Calories: 554 | Fat: 50g | Protein: 20g | Sodium: 773mg | Fiber: 1g | Carbohydrates: 5g | Sugar: 2g

Meaty Zucchini Balls with Yogurt Sauce

Meatballs take on a refreshing flavor with the omission of bread crumbs and the use of bright and flavorful zucchini and mint. Adding a yogurt sauce gives these meatballs an added Mediterranean flair.

Prep Time: 1 hour 15 minutes • Cook Time: 30 minutes

MAKES 12 MEATBALLS

Yogurt Sauce
- ¼ cup sour cream
- ⅓ cup plain yogurt
- ½ tablespoon lemon juice
- 1 medium clove garlic, minced
- 1 tablespoon olive oil
- ¼ teaspoon salt
- ⅛ teaspoon freshly ground black pepper

Meatballs
- 1 large egg
- ½ pound 80/20 ground chuck
- ½ medium zucchini, grated
- 2 green onions, thinly sliced
- 1 tablespoon chopped fresh mint leaves
- 1 tablespoon chopped fresh basil
- 1 large clove garlic, minced
- ½ teaspoon paprika
- ½ teaspoon salt
- ¼ teaspoon cayenne pepper
- ¼ teaspoon freshly ground black pepper
- 1 tablespoon coconut oil

1. Preheat oven to 350°F.
2. Mix all ingredients for yogurt sauce in a small mixing bowl. Chill at least 1 hour.
3. Whisk egg for meatballs in a small bowl. In a separate medium bowl, mix remaining meatball ingredients thoroughly, adding whisked egg last to bind.
4. Form meat mixture into 12 equal balls and place into a muffin tin to bake. Place on top of a cookie sheet and place in oven. Bake meatballs 30 minutes or until meat is browned and internal temperature is at least 165°F.
5. Serve warm with yogurt sauce to dip.

PER 1 MEATBALL WITH DIP Calories: 60 | Fat: 4g | Protein: 4g | Sodium: 81mg | Fiber: 0g | Carbohydrates: 1g | Sugar: 1g

Bacon and Chive Bites

Not all cheesecakes are sweet. With bacon and chives in the mix, this version makes an excellent savory appetizer or midday snack.

Prep Time: 25 minutes • Cook Time: 40–45 minutes

MAKES 6 FAT BOMBS

⅓ cup almond meal flour

1 tablespoon butter, melted

8 ounces cream cheese, softened to room temperature

1 tablespoon bacon grease

1 large egg

4 slices bacon, cooked, cooled, and crumbled into bits

1 large green onion, tops only, thinly sliced

1 medium clove garlic, minced

⅛ teaspoon freshly ground black pepper

Savor the Savory Flavor

Perhaps not as popular, but certainly as delicious, the savory cheesecake makes for an excellent treat. Most savory cakes served in restaurants include flavor combinations such as garlic and Parmesan, bacon and chive, and prosciutto and olive.

1. Preheat oven to 325°F.
2. In a small mixing bowl, combine almond meal and butter.
3. Line 6 cups of a standard-sized muffin tin with cupcake liners. Equally divide flour mixture between cups and press into the bottom gently with the back of a teaspoon. Prebake in oven 10 minutes.
4. While the crust is baking, thoroughly combine cream cheese and bacon grease in a medium mixing bowl with a hand mixer. Add egg and blend until combined.
5. Fold bacon, onion, garlic, and pepper into cheese mixture with a spatula.
6. Divide mixture between prebaked cups, return to oven, and bake another 30–35 minutes until cheese sets. Edges may be slightly browned. To test doneness, insert toothpick into center of cake. If it comes out clean, cheesecake is done.
7. Let cool 5 minutes and serve warm.

PER 1 FAT BOMB Calories: 284 | Fat: 28g | Protein: 7g | Sodium: 297mg | Fiber: 1g | Carbohydrates: 3g | Sugar: 2g

Garlic Pepper Parmesan Crisps

Nothing screams "salty Italian delight!" like Parmesan cheese. Coupled with olive oil, garlic, and a surprise ingredient, these make for a delicious treat by themselves or as a keto-approved cracker for spreads and dips.

Prep Time: 15 minutes • Cook Time: 7–10 minutes

SERVES 2

1 cup shredded Parmesan

¼ teaspoon granulated garlic

¼ teaspoon freshly ground black pepper

1 teaspoon extra-virgin olive oil

1 teaspoon fresh lemon juice

> **Predigested Protein**
> Parmesan cheese is aged so long that much of the protein has already been broken down into peptides and free amino acids before you eat it. This makes digestion easier on you.

1. Preheat oven to 375°F. Prepare a cookie sheet with parchment paper or a Silpat mat.
2. Combine all ingredients in a medium bowl and mix well.
3. Place 2"-wide piles of mixture onto prepared sheet.
4. Bake 7–10 minutes just until edges of cheese start to brown slightly.
5. Let cool 2–3 minutes and remove from sheet with spatula. Can be eaten as is or used as a grain-free alternative in dips or spreads.

PER SERVING Calories: 230 | Fat: 16g | Protein: 20g | Sodium: 897mg | Fiber: 0g | Carbohydrates: 2g | Sugar: 0g

Parmesan Vegetable Crisps

This simple twist on the Parmesan crisp introduces added texture and a mild sweetness while offering additional fiber too. Of course, the added colors of the vegetables make this crisp a beauty for the eyes to feast on before you taste it.

Prep Time: 15 minutes • Cook Time: 7–10 minutes

SERVES 4

¾ cup shredded zucchini

¼ cup shredded carrots

2 cups freshly shredded Parmesan

1 tablespoon olive oil

¼ teaspoon freshly ground black pepper

1. Preheat oven to 375°F. Prepare a cookie sheet with parchment paper or a Silpat mat.
2. Wrap shredded vegetables in a paper towel and wring out excess moisture.
3. Mix all ingredients in a medium bowl until thoroughly combined.
4. Place tablespoon-sized mounds onto prepared cookie sheet.
5. Bake 7–10 minutes until lightly browned.
6. Let cool 2–3 minutes and remove from mat. Enjoy as is or with other fat-bomb dips and spreads.

PER SERVING Calories: 275 | Fat: 18g | Protein: 20g | Sodium: 904mg | Fiber: 0g | Carbohydrates: 3g | Sugar: 1g

Zucchini: A Kitchen Staple

It's no secret that the right vegetables are an important part of any healthy diet. Zucchini is a fantastic choice for high-fat, low-carbohydrate diets because it has a low carbohydrate content (low glycemic index) and it's full of potassium, a crucial mineral for heart health. Besides that, it also makes a fantastic substitute for pasta lovers looking for low-carbohydrate alternatives.

Cheddar Mexi-Melt Crisps

Another versatile cheese for the low-carbohydrate kitchen is Cheddar, the harder the better. Generally the harder Cheddars tend to be the sharpest, so if tart and tangy seems like too much, a mild Cheddar will also work for these crisps.

Prep Time: 15 minutes • Cook Time: 5–7 minutes

SERVES 2

1 cup shredded sharp Cheddar
⅛ teaspoon granulated garlic
⅛ teaspoon chili powder
⅛ teaspoon cumin
1⁄16 teaspoon cayenne pepper (optional)
1 tablespoon finely chopped cilantro
1 teaspoon olive oil

1. Preheat oven to 350°F. Prepare a cookie sheet with parchment paper or a Silpat mat.
2. Mix all ingredients in a medium bowl until well combined.
3. Drop by tablespoon-sized portions onto prepared cookie sheet.
4. Cook 5–7 minutes until edges begin to brown.
5. Allow to cool 2–3 minutes before removing from tray with spatula.
6. Enjoy as is or use as a chip for guacamole.

PER SERVING Calories: 248 | Fat: 21g | Protein: 14g |
Sodium: 353mg | Fiber: 0g | Carbohydrates: 1g | Sugar: 0g

CHAPTER 11

Savory Mousse

Cilantro Mousse

A fresh, tangy, creamy flavor that is totally delicious. Great to pair with the Parmesan Vegetable Crisps (see recipe in Chapter 10).

Prep Time: 6–12 hours • Cook Time: 0 minutes

SERVES 6

2 teaspoons powdered unflavored gelatin

2 tablespoons water

1 ounce sour cream

1 ounce goat cheese, softened

2 tablespoons mayonnaise

3 tablespoons finely chopped fresh cilantro

½ jalapeño pepper, seeded and finely chopped

1 teaspoon lime juice

⅛ teaspoon garlic salt

> **Get Clean with Cilantro**
> Cilantro is highly noted for its ability to act as a natural cleansing agent. The chemical compounds in cilantro bind to toxic metals such as mercury and help remove them from the body. Cilantro also acts as a strong antioxidant and may reduce the risk of heart disease.

1. In a cup, sprinkle gelatin over water and let sit 5 minutes.
2. In a small food processor, mix softened gelatin with remaining ingredients and process until a smooth cream is formed, about 30 seconds.
3. Pour mixture in a large enough mold to hold everything.
4. Refrigerate at least 6 hours or overnight.
5. When ready to eat, dip mold into bowl of hot water to dislodge mousse from container. You can also insert a knife gently between mousse and mold.
6. Invert over a plate and serve.

PER SERVING Calories: 66 | Fat: 6g | Protein: 2g | Sodium: 97mg | Fiber: 0g | Carbohydrates: 1g | Sugar: 0g

Creamy Crab Mousse

This recipe will make a great impression on the guests at your dinner party . . . and they will never know you are serving them a fat bomb.

Prep Time: 6–12 hours • Cook Time: 8 minutes

SERVES 4

1 teaspoon powdered unflavored gelatin
2 tablespoons water
1 ounce cream cheese
1 ounce sour cream
2 tablespoons mayonnaise
2 ounces canned crabmeat, drained
1 tablespoon minced green onion
1 tablespoon minced celery
⅛ teaspoon garlic salt
½ teaspoon lemon juice
⅛ teaspoon freshly ground black pepper

1. In a cup, sprinkle gelatin over water and let sit 5 minutes.
2. In a small saucepan over medium-low heat, melt cream cheese with sour cream. Once melted, add gelatin and mix with a wire whisk until well incorporated.
3. Remove from heat and let cool about 5 minutes.
4. In a medium bowl, mix cream and gelatin with remaining ingredients, blending well.
5. Place crab and cream mixture into a cup-sized mold.
6. Refrigerate at least 6 hours or overnight.
7. When ready to eat, dip mold into bowl of hot water to dislodge mousse from container. You can also insert a knife gently between mousse and mold.
8. Invert over a plate and serve.

PER SERVING Calories: 103 | Fat: 9g | Protein: 4g |
Sodium: 191mg | Fiber: 0g | Carbohydrates: 1g | Sugar: 1g

Creamy Olive Mousse

A wonderful smooth and salty cream that can pair great with any of the cheese crisps in Chapter 10.

Prep Time: 6–12 hours • Cook Time: 0 minutes

SERVES 4

1 tablespoon powdered unflavored gelatin
2 tablespoons hot water
12 large kalamata olives, pitted
4 ounces cream cheese
¼ teaspoon dried parsley flakes
⅛ teaspoon red chili flakes

1. In a cup, dissolve gelatin in water and let sit 5 minutes.
2. In a small food processor, add olives, cream cheese, parsley, chili flakes, and softened gelatin and blend until a very smooth cream is formed.
3. Place mixture in a small serving bowl.
4. Refrigerate at least 6 hours or overnight.
5. Can be refrigerated up to 1 week.

PER SERVING Calories: 108 | Fat: 10g | Protein: 3g | Sodium: 94mg | Fiber: 0g | Carbohydrates: 3g | Sugar: 1g

Gorgonzola Mousse

If you like the pungent flavor of blue cheese, this mousse will quickly become one of your favorites!

Prep Time: 45 minutes • Cook Time: 5–7 minutes

SERVES 4

4 ounces Gorgonzola
1 teaspoon powdered unflavored gelatin
½ cup plus 2 tablespoons heavy whipping cream
⅛ teaspoon freshly ground black pepper

1. Chill a small mixing bowl in the refrigerator.
2. In a small saucepan over medium-low heat, add Gorgonzola and stir until fully melted, about 5 minutes. If clumps remain, you can use an immersion blender to smooth, then remove from heat.
3. Dissolve gelatin in 2 tablespoons cream.
4. Add gelatin to Gorgonzola and mix until well blended.
5. In chilled small bowl, whip ½ cup whipping cream with a hand mixer until stiff peaks form.
6. With a spatula gently fold whipped cream into Gorgonzola.
7. Fill 4 small glasses with mixture and serve with a spoon.
8. Can be refrigerated up to 1 week.

PER SERVING Calories: 234 | Fat: 22g | Protein: 7g |
Sodium: 522mg | Fiber: 0g | Carbohydrates: 2g | Sugar: 0g

Parmesan Mousse

A great mousse to eat by itself or on a cucumber slice. Simple but extremely tasty.

Prep Time: 3 hours 10 minutes • Cook Time: 8 minutes

SERVES 6

2 tablespoons olive oil

1 medium clove garlic, finely minced

1 tablespoon chopped green onion

1 cup heavy cream

1 cup grated Parmesan

> **Hot or Cold?**
> This recipe can be made into a mousse or a hot dip. To turn into a hot dip, place mixture in a small baking dish. Bake at 350°F for 15 minutes until bubbly and browned. Serve with sliced cucumbers or carrots.

1. In a medium heavy-bottomed saucepan, heat olive oil over medium heat. Add green onion and garlic and cook until brown and crispy, about 3 minutes.
2. Add cream and cheese, lower heat, and simmer another 2 minutes, stirring.
3. Remove pot from heat and strain contents though a wide sieve into a bowl so onion solids get filtered out.
4. Let cream come to room temperature, then refrigerate at least 3 hours.
5. Remove from refrigerator and whip with an electric mixer until light and fluffy.
6. Serve immediately.

PER SERVING Calories: 251 | Fat: 24g | Protein: 7g | Sodium: 270mg | Fiber: 0g | Carbohydrates: 2g | Sugar: 0g

Salmon Mousse

This is another recipe you will be proud to serve to your guests—it will make a big impression without a lot of effort on your part. Who said fat bombs can't be shared?

Prep Time: 45 minutes • Cook Time: 0 minutes

SERVES 6

1½ ounces smoked salmon

4 tablespoons mascarpone

2 tablespoons sour cream

1 large hard-boiled egg yolk, put through a fine-mesh strainer

½ tablespoon fresh lemon juice

1 ounce finely chopped chives, plus more for garnish

¼ teaspoon sea salt

¼ teaspoon freshly ground black pepper

2 tablespoons cold whipping cream

6 thin slices cucumber

1. Chop salmon finely with a sharp knife.
2. In a small bowl, beat mascarpone and sour cream with an electric mixer until smooth. Place a second small bowl in refrigerator to chill.
3. Add egg yolk and lemon juice to mascarpone mixture.
4. Add salmon, chives, salt, and pepper to mascarpone mixture and stir well.
5. In previously chilled bowl, whip whipping cream with the electric mixer until stiff peaks form.
6. With a spatula gently fold whipped cream into salmon mixture.
7. Fill 6 small glasses with mixture and serve with a spoon and a slice of cucumber.
8. Can be refrigerated up to 1 week.

PER SERVING Calories: 124 | Fat: 7g | Protein: 5g | Sodium: 208mg | Fiber: 2g | Carbohydrates: 12g | Sugar: 6g

Salmon Sushi Mousse

If you love sushi, this will become your favorite fat bomb. It's super quick and easy to make anytime when that urge for sushi hits.

Prep Time: 8 minutes • Cook Time: 0 minutes

SERVES 6

2 ounces smoked salmon, roughly chopped

2 ounces cream cheese

2 teaspoons wasabi paste

1 teaspoon coconut aminos

6 seaweed snack sheets

> ### Wasabi Paste
> Wasabi is a plant in the same family as horseradish, which is used in Japanese cuisine to accompany sushi dishes. The flavor is similar to horseradish, with a particular pungency that is mainly felt in your nose. Wasabi can be bought in powder and mixed with water to form a paste, or you can buy it directly in paste form ready to use.

1. In a small food processor, add smoked salmon, cream cheese, wasabi, and coconut aminos and blend well until a smooth cream forms.
2. Place 1 tablespoon mixture over each seaweed snack sheet, then roll into a little roll.
3. Serve immediately.

PER SERVING Calories: 50 | Fat: 4g | Protein: 3g | Sodium: 186mg | Fiber: 0g | Carbohydrates: 2g | Sugar: 0g

Shrimp Mousse DF

This recipe makes a great party dish. Just serve with cucumber slices instead of crackers!

Prep Time: 6–12 hours • Cook Time: 0 minutes

SERVES 4

½ tablespoon powdered unflavored gelatin

2 tablespoons hot water

½ cup chopped cooked shrimp

4 ounces coconut cream

½ cup mayonnaise

1 tablespoon chopped green onion

1 tablespoon finely chopped celery

> **Benefits of Shrimp**
> Shrimp is an unusually concentrated source of the carotenoid astaxanthin, which acts as an antioxidant and an anti-inflammatory agent. Shrimp is also an excellent source of the mineral selenium.

1. Dissolve gelatin in hot water and let sit 5 minutes.
2. In a small food processor, add shrimp, coconut cream, mayonnaise, and softened gelatin and blend until a very smooth cream is formed.
3. Move cream from food processor to a bowl, add green onion and celery, and mix well.
4. Place shrimp mixture in a cup-sized mold.
5. Refrigerate at least 6 hours or overnight.
6. When ready to eat, dip mold into bowl of hot water to dislodge mousse from container. You can also insert a knife gently between mousse and mold.
7. Invert over a plate and serve.

PER SERVING Calories: 329 | Fat: 7g | Protein: 7g | Sodium: 233mg | Fiber: 0g | Carbohydrates: 16g | Sugar: 15g

Smoky Deviled Eggs with Riga Sprats Mousse DF

A different take on the usual deviled eggs. This one is chock-full of good fats and quality protein.

Prep Time: 3 hours 10 minutes • Cook Time: 0 minutes

SERVES 4

1 teaspoon powdered unflavored gelatin

2 tablespoons hot water

2 ounces smoked Riga Sprats, drained

2 large hard-boiled eggs, peeled, halved, yolks separated from whites

2 tablespoons olive oil

¼ teaspoon Tabasco

¼ teaspoon sweet paprika

> **Riga Sprats**
> You may never have heard of Riga Sprats, as they are a delicacy imported from Latvia. They are a kind of small, oily fish (*Sprattus sprattus*) from the same family as the sardine. Riga Sprats are smoked and preserved in oil. They are tender and flavorful and make the perfect base for a fat bomb!

1. Dissolve gelatin in hot water and let sit 5 minutes.
2. In a small food processor, add sprats, egg yolks, softened gelatin, olive oil, and Tabasco and blend well until a smooth cream forms.
3. With a spoon, fill mousse into holes of egg whites.
4. Sprinkle with paprika.
5. Refrigerate at least 3 hours before serving.

PER SERVING Calories: 120 | Fat: 11g | Protein: 6g | Sodium: 51mg | Fiber: 0g | Carbohydrates: 0g | Sugar: 0g

Spiced Creamy Chicken Liver Mousse DF

You might not be a big fan of liver, but this recipe could change your mind. The flavor is subtle and creamy and easy to enjoy even for picky eaters.

Prep Time: 6–12 hours • Cook Time: 7 minutes

SERVES 2

3 tablespoons coconut oil, divided
6 ounces fresh chicken livers, cleaned and dried
¼ teaspoon allspice
¼ teaspoon nutmeg
⅛ teaspoon ground cloves
4 ounces coconut cream
2 tablespoons coconut milk
⅛ teaspoon orange zest
⅛ teaspoon sea salt
1 cup cucumber slices

1. In a large heavy-bottomed skillet over medium heat, melt 1 tablespoon coconut oil.
2. Add chicken livers and sauté on high heat on one side without turning until browned on the bottom, about 2 minutes.
3. Flip livers and sprinkle with allspice, nutmeg, and cloves. Sauté until browned, about 3 more minutes.
4. Remove livers from heat and let cool 10 minutes.
5. In a food processor, add chicken livers with all the cooking oil, remaining coconut oil, coconut cream, coconut milk, orange zest, and salt and blend well until a smooth cream forms. For best results use a high-powered blender so the resulting cream will be very smooth.
6. Pour liver cream into 2 ramekins and refrigerate at least 6 hours or overnight.
7. Serve with a spoon and cucumber slices.

PER SERVING Calories: 518 | Fat: 37g | Protein: 16g | Sodium: 231mg | Fiber: 1g | Carbohydrates: 33g | Sugar: 30g

CHAPTER 12

Dressings, Dips, and Spreads

Mojo de Ajo Aioli DF

In Mexican and Latin cuisine, mojo de ajo is considered to be the nectar of the gods. Although it is simple to make, mojo de ajo leaves an everlasting impression on those who've been fortunate enough to taste it.

Prep Time: 1 hour 40 minutes • Cook Time: 1 hour 10 minutes

SERVES 16

1 large head garlic
8 ounces extra-virgin olive oil
¼ teaspoon salt
¼ cup lime juice
1 large egg, at room temperature
⅛ teaspoon cayenne pepper

1. Preheat oven to 325°F.
2. Take garlic head apart and peel individual cloves by slightly smashing each clove with the side of a knife, which makes the papery skin easier to peel.
3. Fill an 8" × 8" glass casserole dish with olive oil, salt, and garlic making sure cloves are fully submerged in the olive oil.
4. Bake 45–50 minutes until garlic is lightly browned. Add lime juice and bake an additional 20 minutes.
5. Remove from oven and let cool.
6. Once at room temperature, smash garlic with fork or potato masher, then add garlic and pour oil into large-mouthed, quart-sized Mason jar.
7. Add egg and cayenne and blend with immersion blender until mixture starts to firm up and turn white, roughly 30 seconds.
8. Place cap on jar and place in refrigerator to firm up for later use as a spread on lettuce wraps or a dip for vegetables.

PER SERVING Calories: 130 | Fat: 14g | Protein: 0g | Sodium: 42mg | Fiber: 0g | Carbohydrates: 1g | Sugar: 0g

Holy Jalapeño Mayonnaise DF

A little bit of heat from the jalapeño gives this mayonnaise just the right amount of kick to a carne asada lettuce wrap or a naked chicken burrito bowl. It also mixes well with salsa to make a delicious dressing for taco salad.

Prep Time: 1 hour 30 minutes • Cook Time: 25 minutes

SERVES 16

1 medium jalapeño
8 ounces extra-virgin olive oil
1 large egg, at room temperature
¼ cup lime juice
¼ teaspoon salt

1. Preheat oven to 400°F.
2. Place jalapeño on a baking sheet and roast until slightly browned, roughly 25 minutes.
3. Let jalapeño cool to room temperature. Once cooled, cut off top, remove ribs and seeds, and finely dice.
4. Pour oil into large-mouthed, quart-sized jar.
5. Add egg, lime juice, and salt and blend with immersion blender until mixture starts to firm up and turn white, roughly 30 seconds.
6. Fold diced pepper into mixture with a small spatula.
7. Place cap on jar and place in refrigerator to firm up for later use as a spread or as a binder for baked and crusted chicken or fish.

PER SERVING Calories: 130 | Fat: 14g | Protein: 0g |
Sodium: 42mg | Fiber: 0g | Carbohydrates: 0g | Sugar: 0g

Simple Keto Mayonnaise DF

One of the problems with traditional store-bought mayonnaise is its reliance on the use of canola, vegetable, and soy oils to keep production costs lower. Make this simple mayonnaise with your choice of the listed oils to keep this fat bomb a healthy option for wraps and salad dressings.

Prep Time: 1 hour 5 minutes • Cook Time: 0 minutes

SERVES 16

8 ounces extra-virgin olive oil, walnut oil, MCT oil, or macadamia oil

1 large egg, at room temperature

2 teaspoons apple cider vinegar

¼ teaspoon salt

⅛ teaspoon freshly ground black pepper

⅛ teaspoon granulated garlic

Benefits of Homemade Mayonnaise

Truly the best way to avoid non-GMO and artery-clogging ingredients in mayonnaise is to simply make it at home. Most commercial production of this condiment includes the use of less expensive corn, soy, and canola oils, which are generally sourced from GMO sources. The use of light-tasting organic oils is a simple and healthy substitution anyone can make.

1. Pour oil into large-mouthed, quart-sized jar.
2. Add egg, vinegar, and spices and blend with immersion blender until mixture starts to firm up and turn white, roughly 20 seconds.
3. Place cap on jar and place in refrigerator to firm up for later use as a versatile spread for wraps, a base for salad dressing, or as a binder for cheese- or nut-crusted fish.

PER SERVING Calories: 128 | Fat: 14g | Protein: 0g | Sodium: 42mg | Fiber: 0g | Carbohydrates: 0g | Sugar: 0g

Lemon Thyme Butter

A simple infusion of lemon and fresh herbs into butter makes it a delicious way to season fish, chicken, seafood, and low-glycemic-index vegetables. While the method to make this butter is easy, it makes the food it flavors taste like a gourmet chef prepared them.

Prep Time: 2 hours • Cook Time: 0 minutes

SERVES 8

8 tablespoons salted butter, at room temperature

2 tablespoons chopped fresh thyme

2 large cloves garlic, peeled

1 tablespoon fresh lemon juice

1. Combine all ingredients in a food processor and pulse to combine.
2. Place mixture in a log shape on a piece of wax paper and twist ends shut.
3. Refrigerate for about 2 hours before use.

PER SERVING Calories: 104 | Fat: 11g | Protein: 0g | Sodium: 82mg | Fiber: 0g | Carbohydrates: 1g | Sugar: 0g

Avocado Mascarpone Butter

This butter works very well on both grilled fish and steak. You can use it whenever you have a lean protein source that you need to add fat to, to achieve your keto requirements. The flavor is very mild and creamy and it will not overpower the flavor of your protein.

Prep Time: 2 hours • Cook Time: 0 minutes

SERVES 10

1 large avocado, pitted and peeled

3 tablespoons butter, softened

¼ teaspoon sea salt

¼ teaspoon freshly ground black pepper

1. Combine all ingredients in a food processor and pulse to combine. Place mixture in a container with an airtight lid.
2. Refrigerate up to 5 days until ready to use.

PER SERVING Calories: 62 | Fat: 6g | Protein: 0g | Sodium: 61mg | Fiber: 1g | Carbohydrates: 2g | Sugar: 0g

Avocado Pecan Dressing DF

This dressing can be used on salads, on shirataki noodles for a pasta salad, on shirataki rice, or even on grilled chicken and fish! The smooth, creamy, and tangy flavor is a nice complement to almost any food.

Prep Time: 35 minutes • Cook Time: 0 minutes

SERVES 16

½ cup pecans

1 tablespoon ½"-sliced green onion

½ cup olive oil

1 small avocado, pitted and peeled

Juice of 1 lime

¼ teaspoon sea salt

2 tablespoons coconut milk

Helpful Prep Tip
To presoak the pecans, just leave out on the counter overnight in warm water and they will be ready to use in the morning.

1. Soak pecans in a cup of warm water 30 minutes, then drain.
2. In a small food processor, add green onion and process until very fine, about 20 seconds.
3. Add pecans and process until almost a cream, about 30 seconds.
4. Add olive oil and process another 30 seconds until well blended.
5. Add avocado, lime juice, salt, and coconut milk.
6. Process about 30–60 seconds until a smooth cream is formed.
7. Transfer to an airtight container. It will keep in the refrigerator about 3 days.

PER SERVING Calories: 108 | Fat: 11g | Protein: 1g | Sodium: 38mg | Fiber: 1g | Carbohydrates: 2g | Sugar: 0g

Hail Caesar Dressing DF

This dairy-free take on the classic dressing is as creamy and delicious as the original version. While a romaine lettuce base is preferred, this dressing also makes an excellent spread inside a grilled chicken lettuce wrap.

Prep Time: 5 minutes • Cook Time: 0 minutes

SERVES 16

½ medium lemon, juiced

½ tablespoon apple cider vinegar

1 large clove garlic, smashed

1 large egg, at room temperature

½ ounce anchovies

¼ teaspoon salt

¼ teaspoon freshly ground black pepper

1 cup extra-virgin olive oil

1. Place all ingredients except oil into a wide-mouthed, quart-sized jar.
2. Blend ingredients with an immersion blender until well chopped and mixed.
3. Add oil and blend 20–30 seconds more until dressing takes on the consistency of thin mayonnaise.
4. Chill until ready to use. Mix before use.

> **How Did Caesar Salad Get Its Name?**
> Despite what many may believe, Caesar salad was not named after the Roman emperor. An Italian-born chef, Caesar Cardini, actually invented the dish in the 1920s with remnants in his restaurant kitchen during a dinner rush. The salad was also served with all the ingredients on individual romaine lettuce leaves and eaten as a finger food.

PER SERVING Calories: 126 | Fat: 14g | Protein: 1g | Sodium: 74mg | Fiber: 0g | Carbohydrates: 0g | Sugar: 0g

Lemon Greek Dressing DF

This dressing showcases lemon as the true star of the show. One taste of this on a romaine lettuce salad topped with kalamata olives is truly what dining in the Greek isles tastes like.

Prep Time: 12 hours • Cook Time: 0 minutes

SERVES 8

4 large cloves garlic

¼ teaspoon salt

½ cup extra-virgin olive oil

2 lemons, juiced

4 tablespoons red wine vinegar

2 tablespoons minced fresh oregano

⅛ teaspoon freshly ground black pepper

A Note on Herbs

You can substitute dried herbs for their fresh counterparts, but keep in mind that dried herbs are more concentrated so they have a stronger flavor. If you choose to use dried herbs instead of fresh, use only ⅓ of the fresh amount. For example, if the recipe calls for 3 tablespoons of fresh herbs, use only 1 tablespoon of dried herbs.

1. Smash garlic cloves with side of knife to remove papery skins. Sprinkle with salt and rub with side of knife to release garlic oils.

2. Place garlic cloves into a pint-sized jar and cover with oil.

3. Add remaining ingredients to jar, tighten lid, and shake to combine.

4. Set in refrigerator overnight in order for flavors to marry. Shake before use. Add more salt to taste if needed.

PER SERVING Calories: 127 | Fat: 14g | Protein: 0g | Sodium: 75mg | Fiber: 0g | Carbohydrates: 2g | Sugar: 0g

Bacon Olive Spread

Bacon and olive are complementary salty flavors that pair well with cream cheese. This spread is great served on celery sticks or cucumber slices.

Prep Time: 8 minutes • Cook Time: 10 minutes

SERVES 4

4 slices bacon
8 ounces cream cheese, softened to room temperature
2 tablespoons olive oil mayonnaise
1 tablespoon freshly squeezed lemon juice
24 Spanish olives, sliced

1. Cook bacon in a large skillet over medium heat until crisp, 5 minutes per side. Drain on paper towel.
2. In a medium mixing bowl, beat softened cream cheese with a hand mixer until smooth.
3. Add mayonnaise and lemon juice and mix on medium speed until combined.
4. Crumble bacon into bowl followed by sliced olives.
5. Fold bacon and olives into cream cheese mixture by hand with rubber spatula.
6. Can be served immediately or cooled in refrigerator to enjoy cold.

PER SERVING Calories: 187 | Fat: 18g | Protein: 3g | Sodium: 319mg | Fiber: 0g | Carbohydrates: 2g | Sugar: 1g

Guacamole Dip DF

The rich and creamy flavors of avocado pair expertly with fresh tomato, onion, and chili peppers. Guacamole makes a fantastic and easy way to add fat to any meal with a Southwestern influence.

Prep Time: 5 minutes • Cook Time: 0 minutes

SERVES 4

1 large avocado, pitted, peeled, and diced

1 tablespoon freshly squeezed lime juice

½ teaspoon salt

2 large cloves garlic, minced

1 small Anaheim chili pepper, diced

½ small yellow onion, peeled and diced

1 small vine-ripened tomato, diced

2 tablespoons freshly chopped cilantro

> **Why Guacamole Is a Superfood**
> Guacamole is full of healthy oleic acid from avocado, proven to help lower harmful LDL cholesterol levels. But what else is so great about it, aside from the taste? With high levels of vitamin K (for increased calcium absorption), vitamin A (which prevents viral and bacterial infections), and lycopene (which reduces the risk of heart disease and cancer), it's a wonder it's not prescribed by doctors.

1. Place avocado in a small bowl along with lime juice, salt, and garlic.
2. Mash avocado slightly with fork or a potato masher.
3. Add chili pepper, onion, tomato, and cilantro and gently fold into mixture.
4. Guacamole can be chilled or served immediately. Pairs well with Cheddar Mexi-Melt Crisps (see recipe in Chapter 10) or as a topping on carne asada wraps.

PER SERVING Calories: 93 | Fat: 7g | Protein: 2g | Sodium: 302mg | Fiber: 4g | Carbohydrates: 7g | Sugar: 2g

Crab Rangoon Dip

Here is one of the best ways to enjoy a Chinese takeout favorite without the added carbohydrates. This dip is best enjoyed on celery sticks or Parmesan crisps.

Prep Time: 10 minutes • Cook Time: 30–35 minutes

SERVES 4

8 ounces cream cheese, softened to room temperature

2 tablespoons olive oil mayonnaise

1 tablespoon freshly squeezed lemon juice

½ teaspoon sea salt

¼ teaspoon freshly ground black pepper

2 medium cloves garlic, minced

2 green onions, diced

½ cup shredded Parmesan

4 ounces canned white crabmeat

> **Allicin and *Allium***
>
> Like shallots, garlic belongs to the genus *Allium*, which also includes onions and leeks. The major compound in garlic, which is called allicin, is responsible for its smell as well as its health benefits, which include boosting the immune system, reducing blood pressure, and reducing the risk of Alzheimer's disease and dementia.

1. Preheat oven to 350°F.
2. In a medium bowl, mix cream cheese, mayonnaise, lemon juice, salt, and pepper with a hand blender until well incorporated.
3. Add garlic, onions, Parmesan, and crabmeat and fold into mixture with a spatula.
4. Transfer mixture to an oven-safe crock and spread out evenly.
5. Bake 30–35 minutes until top of dip is slightly browned. Serve warm.

PER SERVING Calories: 383 | Fat: 32g | Protein: 19g | Sodium: 1,057mg | Fiber: 0g | Carbohydrates: 5g | Sugar: 2g

CHAPTER 13

Classic Sweet Fat Bombs

White Chocolate Pecan Fat Bombs DF

This classic fat-bomb recipe is easy and incredibly delicious. Walnuts would be a great addition if you're out of pecans.

Prep Time: 3 hours • Cook Time: 10 minutes

MAKES 8 FAT BOMBS

¼ cup pecans

4 tablespoons cocoa butter

4 tablespoons coconut oil

¼ teaspoon vanilla extract

5 drops stevia glycerite

> **Be Choosy with Nuts**
> When buying nuts, opt for raw, unsalted varieties rather than roasted, salted, or sugared versions. Raw nuts generally contain no added ingredients, while roasted, flavored nuts can contain unhealthy oils and sugar.

1. Chop pecans coarsely with a knife or process quickly in a food processor so they don't get too fine.
2. In a small saucepan over very low heat, add cocoa butter and coconut oil, stirring until completely melted, about 3 minutes.
3. Remove from heat and stir in pecans, vanilla extract, and stevia.
4. Pour into 8 silicone molds.
5. Refrigerate until hard.
6. Remove from mold. Serve immediately or store in refrigerator for up to 1 week.

PER 1 FAT BOMB Calories: 144 | Fat: 16g | Protein: 0g | Sodium: 0mg | Fiber: 0g | Carbohydrates: 0g | Sugar: 0g

Marzipan Bombs DF

You do not have to be in Germany to enjoy the delicious flavor of marzipan! Make this fat bomb and you will be surprised how much it matches the original flavor.

Prep Time: 3 hours • Cook Time: 0 minutes

MAKES 10 FAT BOMBS
1 cup blanched almonds
3 tablespoons confectioners Swerve
3 tablespoons coconut oil, softened
¼ teaspoon almond extract
1 teaspoon rose water

1. Process almonds and Swerve in a food processor or high-powered blender until they turn into a fine crumble.
2. Add coconut oil, almond, and rose water.
3. Process until mixture starts to ball up and forms a very fine texture.
4. Place into 10 silicone molds.
5. Refrigerate until hard.
6. Remove from mold. Serve immediately or store in refrigerator for up to 1 week.

PER 1 FAT BOMB Calories: 99 | Fat: 9g | Protein: 2g | Sodium: 0mg | Fiber: 1g | Carbohydrates: 4g | Sugar: 3g

Chocolate Peanut Butter Fat Bombs

Chocolate and peanut butter is a combination found in many favorite candies. Get the same delicious flavors here without the guilt of traditional sugary treats.

Prep Time: 3 hours • Cook Time: 10 minutes

MAKES 10 FAT BOMBS

4 tablespoons coconut oil

4 ounces sugar-free baking dark chocolate

¼ cup peanut butter

½ teaspoon vanilla extract

5 drops stevia glycerite

> **Choosing Your Peanut Butter**
>
> When you choose your peanut butter, make sure that it does not contain hydrogenated fats. Also, make sure it does not contain sugar, or hidden sugars like dextrose or sucrose. The best peanut butter you can buy is an all-natural, organic one!

1. In a small saucepan over very low heat, add coconut oil and chocolate, stirring until completely melted, about 3 minutes.
2. Add peanut butter and keep stirring until well blended. If you like a "swirly" effect, use creamy peanut butter and just slightly stir in, leaving it mostly unmixed.
3. Remove from heat and stir in vanilla and stevia.
4. Pour into 8 silicone molds.
5. Refrigerate until hard.
6. Remove from mold. Serve immediately or store in refrigerator for up to 1 week.

PER 1 FAT BOMB Calories: 142 | Fat: 15g | Protein: 3g | Sodium: 32mg | Fiber: 2g | Carbohydrates: 5g | Sugar: 1g

Dark Chocolate Peppermint Fat Bombs

These fat bombs are modeled after the very famous British chocolates After Eight, which are wafer-thin dark chocolates filled with peppermint cream.

Prep Time: 3 hours • Cook Time: 10 minutes

MAKES 8 FAT BOMBS

4 tablespoons coconut oil
4 ounces sugar-free baking dark chocolate
¼ teaspoon peppermint extract
5 drops stevia glycerite

1. In a small saucepan over very low heat, add coconut oil and chocolate, stirring until completely melted, about 3 minutes.
2. Remove from heat and stir in peppermint and stevia.
3. Pour into 8 silicone molds.
4. Refrigerate until hard.
5. Remove from mold. Serve immediately or store in refrigerator for up to 1 week.

PER 1 FAT BOMB Calories: 130 | Fat: 14g | Protein: 2g | Sodium: 3mg | Fiber: 2g | Carbohydrates: 4g | Sugar: 0g

Dark Chocolate Espresso Fat Bombs

Who doesn't love the flavors of chocolate and coffee together? This fat bomb will give you energy without even touching the caffeine!

Prep Time: 3 hours • Cook Time: 7 minutes

MAKES 8 FAT BOMBS

2 tablespoons cocoa butter

2 tablespoons coconut oil

2 ounces sugar-free baking dark chocolate

¼ teaspoon coffee extract

5 drops stevia glycerite

1. In a small saucepan over very low heat, add cocoa butter, coconut oil, and chocolate, stirring until completely melted, about 3 minutes.
2. Remove from heat and stir in coffee extract and stevia.
3. Pour into 8 silicone molds.
4. Refrigerate until hard.
5. Remove from mold. Serve immediately or store in refrigerator for up to 1 week.

PER 1 FAT BOMB Calories: 96 | Fat: 10g | Protein: 1g | Sodium: 2mg | Fiber: 1g | Carbohydrates: 2g | Sugar: 0g

Dark Chocolate Coconut Fat Bombs

A different take on the famous coconut chocolate candy . . . one that is actually good for you!

Prep Time: 3 hours • Cook Time: 7 minutes

MAKES 12 FAT BOMBS

2 tablespoons coconut oil

2 ounces sugar-free baking dark chocolate

1 teaspoon vanilla extract

½ teaspoon coconut extract (optional)

1 tablespoon confectioners Swerve

½ cup shredded unsweetened coconut

1. In a small saucepan over very low heat, add coconut oil, chocolate, extracts, and Swerve, stirring until completely melted, about 3 minutes.
2. Remove from heat and stir in shredded coconut.
3. Pour into 12 silicone molds.
4. Refrigerate until hard.
5. Remove from mold. Serve immediately or store in refrigerator for up to 1 week.

PER 1 FAT BOMB Calories: 58 | Fat: 6g | Protein: 1g | Sodium: 2mg | Fiber: 1g | Carbohydrates: 3g | Sugar: 1g

Chocolate Amaretto Fat Bombs

Have you ever tried the Italian liquor amaretto? These fat bombs will remind you of the delicious flavor but without the alcohol and the sugar.

Prep Time: 3 hours • Cook Time: 7 minutes

MAKES 8 FAT BOMBS
¼ cup almonds
2 tablespoons cocoa butter
2 tablespoons coconut oil
2 ounces sugar-free baking dark chocolate
¼ teaspoon amaretto extract
5 drops stevia glycerite

1. Chop almonds coarsely with a knife or process quickly in a food processor so they don't get too fine.
2. In a small saucepan over very low heat, add cocoa butter, coconut oil, and chocolate, stirring until completely melted.
3. Remove from heat and stir in almonds, amaretto, and stevia.
4. Pour into 8 silicone molds.
5. Refrigerate until hard.
6. Remove from mold. Serve immediately or store in refrigerator for up to 1 week.

PER 1 FAT BOMB Calories: 113 | Fat: 12g | Protein: 2g | Sodium: 2mg | Fiber: 2g | Carbohydrates: 3g | Sugar: 0g

Chocolate Caramel Fat Bombs

This is a creamy, chocolaty fat bomb with the flavor of caramel. The flavor is pretty darn close to candy!

Prep Time: 3 hours • Cook Time: 7 minutes

MAKES 12 FAT BOMBS

6 tablespoons coconut oil

6 tablespoons heavy cream

2 ounces sugar-free baking dark chocolate

2 tablespoons caramel extract

2 tablespoons confectioners Swerve

1. In a small saucepan over very low heat, add coconut oil, cream, chocolate, caramel extract, and Swerve, stirring until completely melted. Pour into 12 silicone molds.
2. Refrigerate until hard. Remove from mold. Serve immediately or store in refrigerator for up to 1 week.

PER 1 FAT BOMB Calories: 120 | Fat: 12g | Protein: 1g | Sodium: 4mg | Fiber: 1g | Carbohydrates: 3g | Sugar: 2g

Coconut Peppermint Fat Bombs DF

You can replace the peppermint extract in this recipe with any other pure extract. Try lemon, orange, almond, or maple.

Prep Time: 30 minutes • Cook Time: 5 minutes

MAKES 12 FAT BOMBS

1 cup coconut butter

¼ cup unsweetened shredded coconut

1 tablespoon coconut oil

½ teaspoon peppermint extract

1. Place all ingredients in a small saucepan over low heat and stir until melted and well combined.
2. Pour an equal amount of mixture into each well of a 12-cup muffin tin lined with cupcake wrappers.
3. Place in freezer and allow to harden, about 30 minutes.
4. Store in refrigerator up to 1 week.

PER 1 FAT BOMB Calories: 176 | Fat: 19g | Protein: 0g | Sodium: 0mg | Fiber: 0g | Carbohydrates: 0g | Sugar: 0g

Almond Butter Fat Bombs

You can replace the almond butter in this recipe with any nut butter of your choice. Cashew butter and peanut butter work really well, too. Just make sure that your nut butter doesn't contain any added sugar.

Prep Time: 35 minutes • Cook Time: 5 minutes

MAKES 12 FAT BOMBS

⅓ cup coconut oil

⅓ cup butter

⅓ cup almond butter

2 tablespoons cream cheese

15 drops liquid stevia

Do It Yourself!

Making your own almond butter is simple and a great way to ensure that it doesn't contain any hidden sugar. Simply put almonds in a food processor and process until the oils break down and a nut butter forms. To up the fat content and make the almond butter smoother, add a couple of teaspoons of almond oil (or another oil of your choice).

1. Place all ingredients in a small saucepan over medium-low heat and stir until melted and mixed together.
2. Pour an equal amount of mixture into each well of a 12-cup silicone mold.
3. Place in freezer until hardened, about 30 minutes.
4. Store in refrigerator up to 1 week.

PER 1 FAT BOMB Calories: 136 | Fat: 14g | Protein: 1g | Sodium: 9mg | Fiber: 0g | Carbohydrates: 3g | Sugar: 2g

Cashew Butter Cup Fat Bombs

Many commercially available cashew butters contain an added sweetener, so be careful when choosing one. If you can't find one at the store, you can always make your own.

Prep Time: 1 hour 10 minutes • Cook Time: 5 minutes

MAKES 12 FAT BOMBS

1 cup coconut oil

¾ cup butter, divided

6 tablespoons cocoa powder

15 drops liquid stevia

¼ cup cashew butter

2 tablespoons heavy whipping cream

> **Nut Butters at Home**
> Making cashew butter is the same basic process as making coconut butter. To make about 1½ cups of cashew butter, place 2 cups unroasted, unsalted cashews in a food processor with a pinch of salt and 1 tablespoon of coconut oil. Process for about 30 seconds and then scrape down the sides of the food processor. Continue processing until smooth, scraping the sides when necessary. Be patient, as the process can take several minutes.

1. Place coconut oil, ½ cup butter, cocoa powder, and stevia in a small saucepan over medium heat and stir until melted and well combined.
2. Pour an equal amount of mixture into each well of a 12-cup mini muffin tin lined with cupcake wrappers. Place muffin tin in freezer and allow to harden, about 30 minutes.
3. Place remaining ¼ cup butter, cashew butter, and whipping cream in a small bowl and beat with a hand mixer until combined and fluffy.
4. Once chocolate mixture in freezer has hardened, spoon an equal amount of cashew butter mixture on top of each well and place in freezer. Allow to harden at least 30 minutes.
5. Store in refrigerator up to 1 week.

PER 1 FAT BOMB Calories: 300 | Fat: 33g | Protein: 1g | Sodium: 5mg | Fiber: 1g | Carbohydrates: 2g | Sugar: 0g

Mixed Nut Bombs

The combination of cashew butter, peanut flour, and almond extract is enough to satisfy every nut lover's craving.

Prep Time: 35 minutes • Cook Time: 0 minutes

MAKES 12 FAT BOMBS

½ cup cashew butter

1 cup defatted unsweetened peanut flour

¼ cup butter, melted

¼ teaspoon almond extract

Defatting Peanuts

Defatted peanut flour is a peanut flour that has had a large percentage of its fat removed through a mechanical process. The fat content of defatted peanut flour still falls around 25 percent of calories, but the shelf life is significantly increased.

1. Mix cashew butter and peanut flour together in a small bowl until well combined.
2. Stir in melted butter until smooth. Add almond extract and stir until combined.
3. Scoop out tablespoons of mixture onto a cookie sheet covered in wax paper.
4. Place in freezer until hardened, about 30 minutes.
5. Store in refrigerator up to 1 week.

PER 1 FAT BOMB Calories: 130 | Fat: 14g | Protein: 1g | Sodium: 2mg | Fiber: 2g | Carbohydrates: 4g | Sugar: 0g

Peanut Butter Cream Cheese Fat Bombs

The crunchy peanut butter and crushed peanuts in this recipe give these peanut butter fat bombs an unbeatable texture. If you prefer less crunch, use smooth peanut butter instead.

Prep Time: 35 minutes • Cook Time: 8 minutes

MAKES 12 FAT BOMBS

1 cup coconut oil
½ cup butter
½ cup crunchy peanut butter
2 tablespoons cream cheese
10 drops liquid stevia
¼ cup crushed unsalted peanuts

1. Place coconut oil, butter, peanut butter, cream cheese, and stevia in a small saucepan over medium heat and stir until melted.
2. Sprinkle crushed peanuts evenly in each well of a 12-cup mini muffin pan lined with cupcake wrappers. Pour peanut butter mixture over peanuts.
3. Place in freezer until hardened, about 30 minutes.
4. Store in refrigerator up to 1 week.

PER 1 FAT BOMB Calories: 316 | Fat: 33g | Protein: 4g | Sodium: 59mg | Fiber: 1g | Carbohydrates: 3g | Sugar: 1g

CHAPTER 14

Sweet Panna Cotta and Custards

Caffè Latte Panna Cotta

Caffè latte is what children have for breakfast in Italy. Isn't this a fun panna cotta?

Prep Time: 6–12 hours • Cook Time: 5 minutes

MAKES 2 FAT BOMBS
½ cup brewed espresso or strong coffee
½ cup heavy whipping cream
1 teaspoon powdered unflavored gelatin
1 tablespoon erythritol or granular Swerve

1. Pour coffee and cream into a small saucepan. Sprinkle gelatin on top and let sit 5 minutes.
2. Add sweetener to saucepan.
3. Place saucepan over low heat and whisk until ingredients are well blended.
4. Simmer on very low heat about 1 minute, stirring constantly.
5. Pour into 2 glasses or molds.
6. Refrigerate until set, at least 6 hours or overnight.
7. Serve in glass or invert over a small plate after dipping glass into hot water a few seconds.

PER 1 FAT BOMB Calories: 211 | Fat: 22g | Protein: 2g | Sodium: 25mg | Fiber: 0g | Carbohydrates: 8g | Sugar: 0g

Indian Basundi Panna Cotta

An exotic dessert from far-away India, with warming spice notes and, of course, delicious creaminess.

Prep Time: 6–12 hours • Cook Time: 10 minutes

MAKES 2 FAT BOMBS

1 cup heavy whipping cream

1 teaspoon powdered unflavored gelatin

1 tablespoon erythritol or granular Swerve

½ teaspoon cardamom

3–4 saffron strands, plus 4 for garnish

2 tablespoons roasted pistachio meat

2 tablespoons coarsely chopped almonds

Saffron

Saffron is a spice derived from the flower of *Crocus sativus*, commonly known as the saffron crocus. The process of harvesting and processing saffron is very labor intensive and the flowers produce very little, making this the most expensive spice in the world. Luckily, a little saffron goes a long way!

1. Pour cream in a small saucepan, sprinkle gelatin on top, and let sit 5 minutes.
2. Add sweetener, cardamom, saffron, and nuts to saucepan.
3. Place saucepan over low heat and whisk until ingredients are well blended.
4. Simmer on very low heat about 5 minutes, stirring constantly.
5. Pour into 2 glasses or molds.
6. Refrigerate until set, at least 6 hours or overnight.
7. Serve in glass or invert over a small plate after dipping glass into hot water a few seconds. Garnish with 2 saffron strands on each fat bomb.

PER 1 FAT BOMB Calories: 360 | Fat: 34g | Protein: 5g | Sodium: 46mg | Fiber: 1g | Carbohydrates: 15g | Sugar: 1g

Lavender Panna Cotta

With the unique and heartwarming essence of lavender, this panna cotta will delight all the senses.

Prep Time: 6–12 hours • Cook Time: 5 minutes

MAKES 2 FAT BOMBS

2 tablespoons plus 1 cup heavy whipping cream, divided
1 teaspoon powdered unflavored gelatin
2 tablespoons plus 1 teaspoon dried lavender, divided
1 tablespoon erythritol or granular Swerve
1 drop lavender essential oil (optional)

1. Place 2 tablespoon cream in a small bowl and sprinkle gelatin on top. Let sit 5 minutes.
2. Pour remaining 1 cup cream in a small saucepan and add 2 tablespoons lavender.
3. Place saucepan over very low heat and stir about 3 minutes. Do not boil. Set aside to rest 10 minutes.
4. Once cream is infused, strain through a fine-mesh sieve.
5. Return saucepan to heat and add softened gelatin and remaining ingredients.
6. Simmer over very low heat about 1 minute, stirring constantly to dissolve gelatin.
7. Pour into 2 glasses or molds.
8. Refrigerate until set, at least 6 hours or overnight.
9. Serve in glass or invert over a small plate after dipping glass into hot water a few seconds. Garnish with ½ teaspoon dried lavender over each fat bomb.

PER 1 FAT BOMB Calories: 469 | Fat: 50g | Protein: 4g | Sodium: 53mg | Fiber: 0g | Carbohydrates: 10g | Sugar: 0g

Meyer Lemon Panna Cotta DF

Tangy and creamy, this is the perfect dessert for a hot summer day.

Prep Time: 6–12 hours • Cook Time: 5 minutes

MAKES 2 FAT BOMBS

1 cup coconut milk
1 teaspoon powdered unflavored gelatin
1 tablespoon erythritol or granular Swerve
Zest of 1 Meyer lemon
1 tablespoon coconut oil
1 teaspoon fresh Meyer lemon juice

1. Pour coconut milk into a small saucepan, sprinkle gelatin on top, and let sit 5 minutes.
2. Add remaining ingredients to saucepan.
3. Place saucepan over low heat and whisk until gelatin and zest are completely incorporated, about 3 minutes.
4. Simmer over very low heat about 1 minute, stirring constantly.
5. Pour into 2 glasses or molds.
6. Refrigerate until set, at least 6 hours or overnight.
7. Serve in glass or invert over a small plate after dipping glass into hot water a few seconds.

PER 1 FAT BOMB Calories: 295 | Fat: 31g | Protein: 4g | Sodium: 18mg | Fiber: 1g | Carbohydrates: 12g | Sugar: 1g

Chocolate Hazelnut Panna Cotta

For any Nutella lover, this hazelnut and chocolate panna cotta will be the ultimate delight, as it has almost no carbs.

Prep Time: 6–12 hours • Cook Time: 8 minutes

MAKES 2 FAT BOMBS

1 cup heavy whipping cream
1 teaspoon powdered unflavored gelatin
4 tablespoons plus 2 teaspoons finely ground hazelnuts, divided
2 tablespoons cocoa powder
1 tablespoon erythritol or granular Swerve
⅛ teaspoon hazelnut flavor

1. Pour cream into a small saucepan, sprinkle gelatin on top, and let sit 5 minutes.
2. In a small nonstick pan over medium heat, toast 4 tablespoons crumbled hazelnuts about 1 minute, stirring constantly. Set aside.
3. Add cocoa powder, sweetener, and hazelnut flavor to cream and gelatin.
4. Place saucepan over low heat and whisk until ingredients are well blended, about 3 minutes.
5. Simmer over very low heat about 1 minute, stirring constantly.
6. Pour into 2 glasses or molds.
7. Refrigerate until set, at least 6 hours or overnight.
8. Serve in glass or invert over a small plate after dipping glass into hot water a few seconds. Garnish with 1 teaspoon crushed hazelnuts over each fat bomb.

PER 1 FAT BOMB Calories: 536 | Fat: 55g | Protein: 7g | Sodium: 49mg | Fiber: 3g | Carbohydrates: 15g | Sugar: 1g

Raspberries and Cream Panna Cotta

A heavenly dream of flavor with real raspberries and cream, sure to uplift anyone's day. Give it a try!

Prep Time: 6–12 hours • Cook Time: 5 minutes

MAKES 2 FAT BOMBS

1 cup heavy whipping cream
1 teaspoon powdered unflavored gelatin
1 tablespoon erythritol or granular Swerve
⅛ teaspoon raspberry flavor
2 tablespoons freeze-dried raspberries

1. Pour cream into a small saucepan, sprinkle gelatin on top, and let sit 5 minutes.
2. Add sweetener and raspberry flavor to saucepan.
3. Place saucepan over low heat and whisk until ingredients are well blended, about 3 minutes.
4. Simmer over very low heat about 1 minute, stirring constantly.
5. Pour into 2 glasses or molds. Sprinkle dried raspberries equally over glasses or molds.
6. Refrigerate until set, at least 6 hours or overnight.
7. Serve in glass or invert over a small plate after dipping glass into hot water a few seconds.

PER 1 FAT BOMB Calories: 434 | Fat: 44g | Protein: 4g | Sodium: 48mg | Fiber: 1g | Carbohydrates: 13g | Sugar: 4g

Turkish Delight Panna Cotta

You will be delighted by the subtle but distinctive flavor of rose petals in this panna cotta. The crunchy pistachios really complete the experience.

Prep Time: 6–12 hours • Cook Time: 5 minutes

MAKES 2 FAT BOMBS

1 cup heavy whipping cream

1 teaspoon powdered unflavored gelatin

1 tablespoon erythritol or granular Swerve

2 tablespoons rose water

2 tablespoons plus 1 teaspoon roasted pistachio meat, divided

> **What Is Turkish Delight?**
> Turkish delight is a family of confections made with starch and sugar. Those are the two things you want to most avoid on a ketogenic diet. But the flavor combination of rose water and crunchy pistachios is always a winner—and makes these fat bombs reminiscent of the original confections.

1. Pour cream into a small saucepan, sprinkle gelatin on top, and let sit 5 minutes.
2. Add sweetener and rose water to saucepan.
3. Place saucepan over low heat and whisk until ingredients are well blended, about 3 minutes.
4. Simmer on very low heat about 1 minute, stirring constantly.
5. Pour into 2 glasses or molds and sprinkle 1 tablespoon pistachios on top of each fat bomb.
6. Refrigerate until set, at least 6 hours or overnight.
7. Serve in glass or invert over a small plate after dipping glass into hot water a few seconds. Garnish each fat bomb with ½ teaspoon roasted pistachios.

PER 1 FAT BOMB Calories: 458 | Fat: 48g | Protein: 5g | Sodium: 105mg | Fiber: 1g | Carbohydrates: 11g | Sugar: 0g

Butterscotch Custard

Silky and sweet with a faint hint of bitter from the butterscotch, this fat bomb could not be more decadent.

Prep Time: 4 hours 15 minutes • Cook Time: 50 minutes

MAKES 2 FAT BOMBS

2 tablespoons unsalted butter
½ cup erythritol or granular Swerve
1 cup heavy cream
2 large egg yolks
1 teaspoon vanilla extract
⅛ teaspoon sea salt

1. Preheat oven to 300°F.
2. Place 2 ramekins in a deep baking pan just large enough to hold them.
3. In a small saucepan over medium heat, melt butter and sweetener and cook until butter browns, about 5 minutes.
4. Very slowly add cream, whisking constantly until completely blended with butter, about 5 minutes.
5. In a small bowl, whisk together remaining ingredients until egg yolks are foamy.
6. Slowly pour egg mixture into cream, whisking constantly to combine well.
7. Pour mixture through a fine strainer into ramekins using a spoon to help you.
8. Pour hot water into baking pan halfway up ramekins.
9. Bake until custard is set, about 35 minutes.
10. Remove from oven and let cool in baking pan about 4 hours.
11. Can be stored in refrigerator up to 3 days.

PER 1 FAT BOMB Calories: 383 | Fat: 40g | Protein: 4g | Sodium: 135mg | Fiber: 0g | Carbohydrates: 35g | Sugar: 0g

Coconut Custard DF

This is a perfect variation of the famous custard, suitable for people with dairy sensitivities. You will find it so delicious, though, that it will become a well-loved recipe for everyone.

Prep Time: 4 hours 15 minutes • Cook Time: 50 minutes

MAKES 2 FAT BOMBS

1 cup coconut cream
1 large egg
1 large egg yolk
½ cup erythritol or granular Swerve
½ teaspoon vanilla extract
½ teaspoon rum extract (optional)

1. Preheat oven to 300°F.
2. Place 2 ramekins in a deep baking pan just large enough to hold them.
3. In a small saucepan over low heat, bring coconut cream to a simmer.
4. In a small bowl, whisk together remaining ingredients until eggs are foamy and sweetener is dissolved.
5. Slowly pour egg mixture into coconut cream, whisking constantly to combine well.
6. Pour mixture through a fine strainer into ramekins using a spoon to help you.
7. Pour hot water into baking pan halfway up ramekins.
8. Bake until custard is set, about 35 minutes.
9. Remove from oven and let cool in baking pan about 4 hours.
10. Can be stored in refrigerator up to 3 days.

PER 1 FAT BOMB Calories: 594 | Fat: 28g | Protein: 6g |
Sodium: 92mg | Fiber: 0g | Carbohydrates: 127g | Sugar: 77g

Creamy Chocolate Custard

Is there such a thing as too much chocolate? Even if you are not a chocolate fan, this unbelievably rich and smooth recipe will make a convert out of you.

Prep Time: 4 hours 15 minutes • Cook Time: 50 minutes

MAKES 2 FAT BOMBS

2 ounces unsweetened baking chocolate

1 cup heavy cream

1 large egg

1 large egg yolk

½ cup erythritol or granular Swerve

1 teaspoon vanilla extract

4 tablespoons unsweetened whipped cream

1. Preheat oven to 300°F.
2. Place 2 ramekins in a deep baking pan just large enough to hold them.
3. In a small saucepan or a double boiler, over very low heat, melt chocolate while slowly stirring.
4. Once chocolate is fluid, very slowly add cream, whisking constantly until it is completely blended with chocolate, about 5 minutes.
5. In a small bowl, whisk egg, egg yolk, sweetener, and vanilla until eggs are foamy and sweetener is dissolved.
6. Slowly pour egg mixture into cream, whisking constantly to combine well. Pour mixture through a fine strainer into ramekins using a spoon to help you.
7. Pour hot water into baking pan halfway up ramekins.
8. Bake until custard is set, about 35 minutes.
9. Remove from oven and let cool in baking pan about 4 hours.
10. Top with whipped cream before serving.
11. Can be stored in refrigerator up to 3 days.

PER 1 FAT BOMB Calories: 473 | Fat: 48g | Protein: 7g | Sodium: 67mg | Fiber: 3g | Carbohydrates: 41g | Sugar: 1g

Espresso Custard

With this recipe you can make your Italian mother-in-law proud!

Prep Time: 4 hours 15 minutes • Cook Time: 50 minutes

MAKES 2 FAT BOMBS

1 cup heavy cream
¼ cup very strong brewed espresso
1 large egg
1 large egg yolk
½ cup erythritol or granular Swerve
1 teaspoon coffee extract (optional)

1. Preheat oven to 300°F.
2. Place 2 ramekins in a deep baking pan just large enough to hold them.
3. In a small saucepan over low heat, bring cream and espresso to a simmer.
4. In a small bowl, whisk together remaining ingredients until eggs are foamy and sweetener is dissolved.
5. Slowly pour egg mixture into cream, whisking constantly to combine well.
6. Pour mixture through a fine strainer into ramekins using a spoon to help you.
7. Pour hot water into baking pan halfway up ramekins.
8. Bake until custard is set, about 35 minutes.
9. Remove from oven and let cool in baking pan about 4 hours.
10. Can be stored in refrigerator up to 3 days.

PER 1 FAT BOMB Calories: 476 | Fat: 49g | Protein: 7g |
Sodium: 85mg | Fiber: 0g | Carbohydrates: 52g | Sugar: 0g

Simple Custard

Custard is a classic dessert with a mild yet sophisticated flavor. Both kids and adults will love this fat bomb.

Prep Time: 4 hours 15 minutes • Cook Time: 50 minutes

MAKES 2 FAT BOMBS

1 cup heavy cream
1 large egg
1 large egg yolk
½ cup erythritol or granular Swerve
1 teaspoon vanilla extract

1. Preheat oven to 300°F.
2. Place 2 ramekins in a deep baking pan just large enough to hold them.
3. In a small saucepan over low heat, bring cream to a simmer.
4. In a small bowl, whisk together remaining ingredients until eggs are foamy and sweetener is dissolved.
5. Slowly pour egg mixture into cream, whisking constantly to combine well.
6. Pour mixture through a fine strainer into ramekins using a spoon to help you.
7. Pour hot water into baking pan halfway up ramekins.
8. Bake until custard is set, about 35 minutes.
9. Remove from oven and let cool in baking pan about 4 hours.
10. Can be stored in refrigerator up to 3 days.

PER 1 FAT BOMB Calories: 482 | Fat: 49g | Protein: 7g |
Sodium: 85mg | Fiber: 0g | Carbohydrates: 52g | Sugar: 1g

CHAPTER 15

Truffles, Fudge, and Bark

Coconut Almond Truffles

The flavors in this recipe are reminiscent of the famous candy bar. This fat bomb really tastes like the original!

Prep Time: 2 hours 10 minutes • Cook Time: 20 minutes

MAKES 12 FAT BOMBS

Ganache

2 ounces cocoa butter

2 ounces coconut cream

2 tablespoons confectioners Swerve

2 drops stevia glycerite

4 tablespoons unsweetened shredded coconut

12 whole almonds

Coating

3 ounces unsweetened chocolate chips

3 tablespoons coarsely chopped almonds

1. In a small double boiler (bain-marie) over medium-low heat, melt cocoa butter slowly, stirring often.
2. Add coconut cream, Swerve, stevia, and shredded coconut and mix well until incorporated.
3. Remove from heat and keep stirring about 10 seconds.
4. Let cool at room temperature until ganache mix solidifies.
5. As soon as the ganache is solid enough to shape, form into 12 balls, place an almond in center of each ball, and wrap ganache mix around almonds. Refrigerate at least 1 hour until very firm.
6. In a small double boiler over medium-low heat, melt chocolate chips. Dip each ganache ball into chocolate coating with a fork or long toothpick to evenly cover.
7. Place chopped almonds on a medium plate and roll truffles through until lightly coated. Place coated truffles on a cookie sheet and refrigerate until hard and ready to eat.

PER 1 FAT BOMB Calories: 120 | Fat: 11g | Protein: 2g |
Sodium: 4mg | Fiber: 2g | Carbohydrates: 7g | Sugar: 4g

Dark Chocolate Orange Truffles

The flavor combination of orange and dark chocolate is sometimes called Martinique, especially as an ice cream flavor. It is a delicious combination that can inspire you to dream of faraway resorts.

Prep Time: 1 hour 15 minutes • Cook Time: 10 minutes

MAKES 9 FAT BOMBS

Ganache

3 ounces unsweetened baking chocolate
2 tablespoons heavy cream
1 tablespoon butter
2 tablespoons confectioners Swerve
2 drops stevia glycerite
½ teaspoon liquid orange flavor

Coating

1 teaspoon confectioners Swerve
2 teaspoons unsweetened cocoa powder
1 teaspoon fresh orange zest

Food Flavoring

Using the best-quality food flavors is important for your health! Make sure you get organic and all-natural flavors, without artificial coloring or chemical additives. See Appendix B for a complete list of keto-approved foods.

1. In a small double boiler (bain-marie) over medium-low heat, melt chocolate while slowly stirring.
2. Add cream, butter, Swerve, stevia, and orange flavor to chocolate and mix well until incorporated.
3. Remove from heat and keep stirring about 10 seconds.
4. Place saucepan in refrigerator about 1 hour until ganache has solidified.
5. Scoop ganache with a spoon and form 9 little balls. You might want to wear plastic gloves to help the chocolate not stick to your hands.
6. To make coating, mix confectioners Swerve, cocoa powder, and orange zest on a medium plate. Roll ganache balls through coating powder until thinly coated.
7. For best consistency, keep refrigerated if room temperature exceeds 70°F.

PER 1 FAT BOMB Calories: 78 | Fat: 7g | Protein: 1g |
Sodium: 4mg | Fiber: 2g | Carbohydrates: 5g | Sugar: 2g

Dark Chocolate Raspberry Truffles

A delightful mix of sweet raspberry flavor and bitter dark chocolate—what a heavenly combination!

Prep Time: 1 hour 10 minutes • Cook Time: 10 minutes

MAKES 9 FAT BOMBS

Ganache

3 ounces unsweetened baking chocolate

2 tablespoons heavy cream

1 tablespoon butter

2 tablespoons confectioners Swerve

2 drops stevia glycerite

½ teaspoon liquid raspberry flavor

Coating

3 tablespoons crushed freeze-dried raspberries

Freeze-Dried Raspberries

Freeze-dried raspberries are a genius invention for cooking. They are relatively low in carbohydrates for a fruit and give a big punch of flavor.

1. In a small double boiler (bain-marie) over medium-low heat, melt chocolate while slowly stirring.
2. Add cream, butter, Swerve, stevia, and raspberry flavor to chocolate and mix well until incorporated.
3. Remove from heat and keep stirring about 10 seconds.
4. Place saucepan in refrigerator about 1 hour until ganache has solidified.
5. Scoop ganache with a spoon and form 9 little balls. You might want to wear plastic gloves to help the chocolate not stick to your hands.
6. Place crushed raspberries on a medium plate and roll truffles through until thinly coated.
7. For best consistency, keep refrigerated if room temperature exceeds 70°F.

PER 1 FAT BOMB Calories: 82 | Fat: 7g | Protein: 1g | Sodium: 4mg | Fiber: 2g | Carbohydrates: 6g | Sugar: 3g

Hazelnut Truffles

These truffles have the flavoring of your favorite hazelnut spread, and are just as delicious as the real thing.

Prep Time: 1 hour 10 minutes • Cook Time: 10 minutes

MAKES 9 FAT BOMBS

Ganache

2 ounces unsweetened baking chocolate

1 tablespoon butter

1 tablespoon cream cheese

3 tablespoons finely chopped toasted hazelnuts

2 tablespoons confectioners Swerve

2 drops stevia glycerite

½ teaspoon liquid hazelnut flavor

½ teaspoon sea salt

Coating

3 tablespoons finely chopped toasted hazelnuts

> **Balls or Shapes?**
> You can use fun silicone molds to make your truffles into shapes like hearts or seashells. Just pour the ganache straight from the saucepan into the molds and then refrigerate until solid. When ready, remove from the mold and roll into coating agent.

1. In a small double boiler (bain-marie) over medium-low heat, melt chocolate while slowly stirring.
2. Add butter, cream cheese, hazelnuts, Swerve, stevia, and hazelnut flavor to chocolate and mix well until incorporated.
3. Remove from heat and keep stirring about 10 seconds.
4. Cool at room temperature about 1 hour until ganache has solidified.
5. Scoop ganache with a spoon and form 9 little balls. You might want to wear plastic gloves to help the chocolate not stick to your hands.
6. Place chopped hazelnuts on a medium plate and roll truffles through to coat evenly.

PER 1 FAT BOMB Calories: 85 | Fat: 8g | Protein: 2g | Sodium: 138mg | Fiber: 1g | Carbohydrates: 4g | Sugar: 2g

Salted Caramel and Pecan Truffles

This truffle is a quite indulgent one. Keep it for those moments when you feel you need a special treat.

Prep Time: 1 hour 10 minutes • Cook Time: 10 minutes

MAKES 9 FAT BOMBS

Ganache
2 ounces unsweetened baking chocolate
1 tablespoon butter
1 tablespoon cream cheese
2 tablespoons confectioners Swerve
2 drops stevia glycerite
½ teaspoon liquid caramel flavor
½ teaspoon sea salt

Coating
3 tablespoons chopped pecans

1. In a small double boiler (bain-marie) over medium-low heat, melt chocolate while slowly stirring.
2. Add butter, cream cheese, Swerve, stevia, caramel flavor, and salt to chocolate and mix well until incorporated.
3. Remove from heat and keep stirring about 10 seconds.
4. Place saucepan in refrigerator about 1 hour until ganache has solidified.
5. Scoop ganache with a spoon and form 9 little balls. You might want to wear plastic gloves to help the chocolate not stick to your hands.
6. Place chopped pecans on a medium plate and roll truffles through to coat evenly.

PER 1 FAT BOMB Calories: 83 | Fat: 7g | Protein: 1g | Sodium: 137mg | Fiber: 1g | Carbohydrates: 4g | Sugar: 2g

Smoky Spicy Dark Chocolate Truffles

The sharp flavor of dark chocolate blends incredibly well with the smokiness of chipotle, giving this truffle an exotic flavor reminiscent of the ancient Mayas and Mexico.

Prep Time: 1 hour 10 minutes • Cook Time: 10 minutes

MAKES 9 FAT BOMBS

Ganache

3 ounces unsweetened baking chocolate
2 tablespoons heavy cream
1 tablespoon butter
2 tablespoons confectioners Swerve
2 drops stevia glycerite
½ teaspoon smoked chipotle powder

Coating

1 teaspoon confectioners Swerve
2 teaspoons unsweetened cocoa powder
½ teaspoon smoked chipotle powder

1. In a small double boiler (bain-marie) over medium-low heat, melt chocolate while slowly stirring.
2. Add cream, butter, Swerve, stevia, and chipotle powder to chocolate and mix well until incorporated.
3. Remove from heat and keep stirring about 10 seconds.
4. Place saucepan in refrigerator about 1 hour until ganache has solidified.
5. Scoop ganache with a spoon and form 9 little balls. You might want to wear plastic gloves to help the chocolate not stick to your hands.
6. Mix coating ingredients together in a small bowl.
7. Roll ganache balls into coating powder until thinly coated.
8. For best consistency keep refrigerated for up to 1 week.

PER 1 FAT BOMB Calories: 79 | Fat: 7g | Protein: 1g |
Sodium: 7mg | Fiber: 2g | Carbohydrates: 5g | Sugar: 2g

Almond Pistachio Fudge

This delightful fudge is full of nutty goodness. The addition of firm coconut oil and coconut milk helps give this fudge body and texture.

Prep Time: 4 hours 15 minutes • Cook Time: 5 minutes

MAKES 12 FAT BOMBS

¼ cup cocoa butter

½ cup almond butter

½ cup coconut oil

¼ cup canned coconut milk, chilled overnight

2 tablespoons ghee

2 teaspoons vanilla extract

⅛ teaspoon salt

¼ cup chopped pistachios

> **Pistachios, the Festive Nut**
>
> Bright green colored and delicious, this nut is often reserved for holiday parties—probably due to their higher price. Oddly enough, until the 1980s, manufacturers followed the widespread practice of dying the nuts red! Always opt for naturally colored and roasted nuts for the freshest flavor, and to avoid any additives or dyes.

1. Grease and line an 8" × 8" baking pan with parchment paper.

2. Melt cocoa butter in a small saucepan over low heat and set aside.

3. In a large bowl, add all ingredients except nuts and melted cocoa butter. Mix with a hand mixer until texture is fluffy.

4. Pour melted cocoa butter into almond mixture and combine with hand mixer on low speed.

5. Spread mixture evenly into pan and sprinkle with pistachios.

6. Refrigerate at least 4 hours to set. Cut into 12 bars and serve from refrigerator.

PER 1 FAT BOMB Calories: 228 | Fat: 23g | Protein: 3g | Sodium: 75mg | Fiber: 1g | Carbohydrates: 3g | Sugar: 1g

Brown Butter Rum Pecan Fudge

Browning the butter before making this fudge gives it an extra richness and a gorgeous color. The addition of rum extract makes this fudge's flavor a throwback to vintage butter rum hard candies.

Prep Time: 2 hours 35 minutes • Cook Time: 8 minutes

MAKES 6 FAT BOMBS

8 tablespoons butter
2 ounces cream cheese
½ cup peanut butter
1 teaspoon rum extract
16 drops liquid stevia
¼ cup chopped pecans

1. Grease and line an 8" × 8" baking pan with parchment paper.
2. In a small saucepan over medium-low heat, melt butter until it begins to brown slightly, then add cream cheese and stir to combine.
3. Add peanut butter, rum extract, and liquid stevia and stir until melted and well combined.
4. Stir pecans into mixture and spread into baking dish.
5. Allow to cool to room temperature, then place in refrigerator to finish setting, about 2 hours. Slice into 6 pieces to serve.

PER 1 FAT BOMB Calories: 327 | Fat: 33g | Protein: 7g | Sodium: 131mg | Fiber: 2g | Carbohydrates: 5g | Sugar: 3g

Caramel Coffee Fudge

Sweet coffee and cream is such a treat. Adding an extra kick of caramel flavor gives this fudge the taste of a fancy coffee delivered by a barista, but better. This version is full of fat and none of the sugar.

Prep Time: 1 hour 30 minutes • Cook Time: 10 minutes

MAKES 6 FAT BOMBS

2 tablespoons butter

½ cup heavy cream

2 tablespoons granular Swerve

1 tablespoon instant coffee granules

1. In a small saucepan over medium heat, add all ingredients except coffee.
2. Heat and stir well to combine. Allow to bubble an additional 2–3 minutes.
3. Add coffee granules and stir.
4. Pour mixture into 6 silicone candy molds or into a silicone-bottomed ice cube tray.
5. Allow to cool to room temperature. Place in refrigerator an additional 1 hour to set.

PER 1 FAT BOMB Calories: 103 | Fat: 11g | Protein: 0g | Sodium: 8mg | Fiber: 0g | Carbohydrates: 1g | Sugar: 0g

Chocolate Walnut Fudge

The rich and creamy texture of this chocolate fudge is intensified by using black walnuts. Truthfully, any old walnut will do for this goodie, as long as it's fresh!

Prep Time: 2 hours 35 minutes • Cook Time: 8 minutes

MAKES 4 FAT BOMBS

8 tablespoons butter

4 ounces cream cheese, softened

3 tablespoons cocoa powder

2 tablespoons granular Swerve

1 tablespoon vanilla extract

¼ cup walnut pieces

1. Grease and line a 9" × 5" loaf pan with parchment paper.
2. In a medium saucepan over medium-low heat, melt butter. Add cream cheese and stir until well melted and combined.
3. Remove from heat and add remaining ingredients except walnuts. Mix well.
4. Fold in walnuts and then spread mixture into lined loaf pan.
5. Let cool to room temperature, then place in refrigerator to finish setting, at least 2 hours.
6. Slice into 4 pieces before serving.

PER 1 FAT BOMB Calories: 365 | Fat: 37g | Protein: 4g | Sodium: 94mg | Fiber: 2g | Carbohydrates: 5g | Sugar: 2g

Eggnog Fudge

Nothing says holidays like the creamy, old-fashioned flavor of egg-nog. While an excellent fat bomb on its own, eggnog is usually full of too much sugar to make it a worthwhile treat for a low-carb, high-fat dieter. Now you can enjoy the flavor of the holidays without the sugar overload.

Prep Time: 2 hours 30 minutes • Cook Time: 10 minutes

MAKES 4 FAT BOMBS

8 tablespoons butter

4 ounces cream cheese, softened

1 tablespoon vanilla extract

1 teaspoon nutmeg

¼ teaspoon cinnamon

⅛ teaspoon ground cloves

2 tablespoons granular Swerve

How Did Eggnog Get Its Name?

While the origin of the drink is still up for debate, the name "eggnog" most likely comes from the small wooden cup it was originally served in, known as a noggin.

1. Grease and line a 9" × 5" loaf pan with parchment paper.
2. In a medium saucepan over medium-low heat, melt butter. Add cream cheese and stir until well melted and combined.
3. Remove from heat, add remaining ingredients, and mix well.
4. Spread mixture into lined loaf pan.
5. Let cool to room temperature, then place in refrigerator to finish setting, at least 2 hours.
6. Slice into 4 pieces before serving.

PER 1 FAT BOMB Calories: 312 | Fat: 32g | Protein: 2g | Sodium: 94mg | Fiber: 0g | Carbohydrates: 2g | Sugar: 1g

Maple Bacon Fudge DF

Many low-carb, high-fat dieters love breakfast but miss breakfast cakes covered in maple syrup. This fudge is the one to make for those who long for sugar- and gluten-filled waffles, with a side of bacon included.

Prep Time: 1 hour 5 minutes • Cook Time: 5 minutes

MAKES 12 FAT BOMBS

¼ cup almond butter

¼ cup coconut oil

¼ cup bacon grease, strained

½ teaspoon maple extract

12 drops liquid stevia

2 tablespoons cocoa powder

2 strips cooked bacon, cut into bits

> **Nitrate-Free Bacon**
> Bacon is a natural treasure. Many people are surprised to realize they can actually lose weight while eating bacon on a low-carb, high-fat diet. Fortunately, there are many varieties of bacon available without nitrates (nitrates can cause many health problems).

1. Heat a medium saucepan over medium heat and add almond butter, coconut oil, and bacon grease, stirring until melted.
2. Once melted, add maple, stevia, and cocoa powder. Stir well to combine. Add bacon and stir.
3. Pour mixture into 12 slots in a silicone candy mold or silicone-bottomed ice cube tray.
4. Refrigerate at least 1 hour until set.

PER 1 FAT BOMB Calories: 100 | Fat: 10g | Protein: 2g | Sodium: 72mg | Fiber: 1g | Carbohydrates: 2g | Sugar: 1g

Matcha Berry Fudge

Matcha introduced into this fudge gives it a fresh yet sweet taste. The beautiful color contrasts nicely with fresh or freeze-dried raspberries for a visual treat while you eat.

Prep Time: 4 hours 10 minutes • Cook Time: 5 minutes

MAKES 8 FAT BOMBS

¼ cup cocoa butter

½ cup almond butter

2 tablespoons ghee or butter

2 tablespoons coconut oil

⅓ cup canned coconut milk

2 tablespoons matcha (green tea powder)

1 teaspoon vanilla extract

1 tablespoon granular Swerve

2 tablespoons freeze-dried raspberries

> **What's So Special about Matcha?**
> Some of the many benefits of this antioxidant-rich powdered tea originating from Japan include enhanced energy, better concentration, and more endurance. In addition, this powder is said to lower cholesterol levels, detoxify the liver, burn calories, and enhance calmness.

1. Grease and line a 9" × 5" loaf pan with parchment paper.
2. Melt cocoa butter, almond butter, ghee, and coconut oil over medium-low heat in a medium saucepan. Remove from heat and cool about 5 minutes.
3. Mix in remaining ingredients except raspberries.
4. Pour mixture into lined loaf pan. Sprinkle with raspberries.
5. Place in refrigerator and allow to set at least 4 hours. Slice into 8 pieces before serving.

PER 1 FAT BOMB Calories: 260 | Fat: 29g | Protein: 0g | Sodium: 1mg | Fiber: 0g | Carbohydrates: 1g | Sugar: 0g

Orange Cream Fudge

Orange brightens the flavor of this thick and creamy fudge. Although using juice from a freshly squeezed orange is recommended, use of orange extract would work in a pinch while lowering the carbohydrate count of this treat as well.

Prep Time: 2 hours 10 minutes • Cook Time: 8 minutes

MAKES 4 FAT BOMBS

8 tablespoons butter

4 ounces cream cheese, softened

2 tablespoons freshly squeezed orange juice

1 tablespoon orange zest

½ teaspoon vanilla extract

1. Grease and line a 9" × 5" loaf pan with parchment paper.
2. In a medium saucepan over medium-low heat, melt butter. Add cream cheese and stir until well melted and combined.
3. Remove from heat, add remaining ingredients, and mix well.
4. Spread mixture into lined loaf pan.
5. Let cool to room temperature, then place in refrigerator to finish setting, at least 2 hours.
6. Slice into 4 pieces before serving.

PER 1 FAT BOMB Calories: 305 | Fat: 33g | Protein: 2g | Sodium: 93mg | Fiber: 0g | Carbohydrates: 2g | Sugar: 2g

Peanut Butter Fudge DF

The simple flavors of peanut butter, vanilla, and coconut make this fudge a delicious alternative to many of the chocolate-based fudges. This fudge also sets quickly and can be consumed in less than 30 minutes if chilled in the freezer to accelerate the setting process.

Prep Time: 35 minutes • Cook Time: 5 minutes

MAKES 12 FAT BOMBS
⅔ cup almond butter
⅓ cup coconut oil
1 tablespoon vanilla extract
8 drops liquid stevia

1. Heat a small saucepan over medium heat. Add almond butter and coconut oil and melt.
2. Once melted, add vanilla and stevia and stir well to combine.
3. Pour mixture into 12 slots in a silicone candy mold or silicone-bottomed ice cube tray.
4. Refrigerate 30 minutes until set.

PER 1 FAT BOMB Calories: 163 | Fat: 18g | Protein: 3g | Sodium: 2mg | Fiber: 2g | Carbohydrates: 4g | Sugar: 0g

Salty Peanut Butter Cup Fudge DF

The simple addition of coarse sea salt elevates this fudge to the flavor of a very popular American candy treat. While the cup version of this delicacy is full of sugar and contains dairy, this fudge will satisfy any dairy-free, low-carb, high-fat dieter's sweet tooth.

Prep Time: 2 hours 5 minutes • Cook Time: 8 minutes

MAKES 12 FAT BOMBS

½ cup almond butter

½ cup coconut oil

12 drops liquid stevia

3 tablespoons cocoa powder

1 tablespoon vanilla extract

1 teaspoon coarse sea salt

Popularity of the Peanut Butter in Reese's Cups

Many consumers of Reese's Peanut Butter Cups find the taste of the salty filling irreplaceable. Though you can't buy that filling, consumers can buy Reese's branded peanut butter. In the 1990s, Hershey's released their line of Reese's Peanut Butter to compete with the likes of Skippy and Jif. Those following a ketogenic diet should opt to use natural peanut butters instead.

1. Heat a small saucepan over medium heat. Add almond butter and coconut oil and melt.
2. Once melted, add stevia, cocoa powder, and vanilla and stir well to combine.
3. Pour mixture into 12 slots in a silicone candy mold or silicone-bottomed ice cube tray.
4. Sprinkle coarse sea salt on top of each fat bomb.
5. Refrigerate at least 2 hours until set.

PER 1 FAT BOMB Calories: 150 | Fat: 15g | Protein: 3g | Sodium: 246mg | Fiber: 1g | Carbohydrates: 3g | Sugar: 1g

Toasted Coconut Bark DF

Although delicious with regular shredded coconut, toasting the shaved coconut meat adds an extra nutty flavor that's hard to beat. The addition of another tropical nut elevates this bark to divine.

Prep Time: 2 hours • Cook Time: 10 minutes

SERVES 12

⅓ cup coconut flakes

1 cup coconut oil

¼ cup confectioners Swerve

⅔ cup coarsely chopped macadamia nuts

> **Macadamia Madness**
> Macadamia nuts have grown so much in popularity that California decided to get in on the growing action in the late 1980s. While the trees take 4–5 years to produce the nuts, they were an excellent investment for the warm climate in the southwestern states. Hawaii, however, is still the largest producer of these tasty nuts.

1. Line an 8" × 8" pan with parchment paper.
2. In a small nonstick pan over medium heat, toast coconut flakes just until meat turns light brown. Set aside.
3. Combine coconut oil and sweetener in a small pot over medium heat, stirring frequently until melted. Turn off heat.
4. Add coconut flakes and nuts to pan and stir.
5. Pour mixture into lined pan and spread out with the back of a wooden spoon.
6. Freeze or refrigerate to set bark.
7. Break bark into chunks before serving.

PER SERVING Calories: 244 | Fat: 27g | Protein: 1g | Sodium: 2mg | Fiber: 1g | Carbohydrates: 2g | Sugar: 1g

Blueberry Almond Butter Bark DF

Rich almond butter plays well against the subtle sweetness of fresh blueberries in this bark. Frozen or freeze-dried blueberries would also make an excellent substitute if blueberries are out of season.

Prep Time: 2 hours • Cook Time: 8 minutes

SERVES 12

½ cup almond butter
½ cup coconut oil
12 drops liquid stevia
½ teaspoon vanilla extract
½ cup fresh blueberries

1. Line an 8" × 8" pan with parchment paper.
2. Combine almond butter, coconut oil, stevia, and vanilla in a small saucepan over medium heat, stirring frequently until ingredients have melted.
3. Add blueberries and simmer 2–3 minutes more.
4. Pour mixture into lined pan.
5. Freeze or refrigerate to set bark.
6. Break bark into chunks before serving.

PER SERVING Calories: 147 | Fat: 15g | Protein: 3g |
Sodium: 49mg | Fiber: 1g | Carbohydrates: 3g | Sugar: 2g

Strawberry White Chocolate Bark DF

Tart berries make an excellent partner with sweet white chocolate. While this recipe uses fresh strawberries, it would taste just as good with fresh or frozen raspberries, blackberries, or cherries.

Prep Time: 2 hours • Cook Time: 8 minutes

SERVES 12

¼ cup coconut butter
½ cup coconut oil
1 teaspoon vanilla extract
2 tablespoons confectioners Swerve
½ cup diced fresh strawberries

1. Line an 8" × 8" pan with parchment paper.
2. Combine coconut butter, coconut oil, vanilla, and Swerve in a small saucepan over medium heat, stirring frequently until ingredients have melted.
3. Turn off heat and stir in strawberries.
4. Pour mixture into lined pan.
5. Freeze or refrigerate to set bark.
6. Break bark into chunks before serving.

Is White Chocolate Actually Chocolate?
Truth be told, white chocolate isn't actually chocolate at all because it is missing the key ingredient, cocoa solids, otherwise thought of as cocoa, like in cocoa powder. However, the cocoa butter that is present in white chocolate is what often keeps the name "chocolate" in this white sweet treat's name.

PER SERVING Calories: 128 | Fat: 14g | Protein: 0g | Sodium: 0mg | Fiber: 0g | Carbohydrates: 2g | Sugar: 2g

Salted Pecan Brittle Bark

Brittle is a delicious and easy-to-make bark. The subtle sweetness of the pecans in this bark will truly make peanut brittle a distant memory to most taste buds.

Prep Time: 2 hours • Cook Time: 8 minutes

SERVES 8

¼ cup butter
¼ cup confectioners Swerve
2 teaspoons vanilla extract
1 cup whole pecans
⅛ teaspoon coarse sea salt

1. Line an 8" × 8" pan with parchment paper.
2. Combine butter, Swerve, and vanilla in a small saucepan over medium heat, stirring frequently until ingredients have melted.
3. Add pecans and bring mixture to a boil, stirring constantly. Cook 2–3 minutes more until mixture is golden brown.
4. Pour mixture into lined pan. Spread out with the back of a wooden spoon and sprinkle with sea salt.
5. Freeze or refrigerate to set bark.
6. Break bark into chunks before serving.

PER SERVING Calories: 148 | Fat: 16g | Protein: 1g |
Sodium: 38mg | Fiber: 1g | Carbohydrates: 2g | Sugar: 1g

Chocolate Pistachio Bark DF

This bark makes a great holiday present. Make large batches and give to your family or coworkers to enjoy.

Prep Time: 2 hours • Cook Time: 5 minutes

SERVES 8

½ cup coconut oil

¼ cup confectioners Swerve

⅓ cup cocoa powder

⅓ cup roughly chopped pistachios

1. Line an 8" × 8" pan with parchment paper.
2. Combine coconut oil and sweetener in a small pot over medium heat, stirring frequently until ingredients have melted.
3. Add cocoa and mix well. Remove from heat.
4. Pour mixture into lined pan. Sprinkle pistachios on top of chocolate layer.
5. Freeze or refrigerate to set bark.
6. Break bark into chunks before serving.

PER SERVING Calories: 342 | Fat: 34g | Protein: 5g | Sodium: 3mg | Fiber: 6g | Carbohydrates: 12g | Sugar: 1g

Chocolate and Nuts, a Lifelong Pair

Does it seem like these two ingredients are lifetime partners? Candy makers in the know have made chocolate-covered nuts, or nut bars, part of their repertoire for over a century. So if it seems like peanuts, almonds, pecans, and cashews have been paired with chocolate for ages, it's because they have. Why mess with a winning recipe?

CHAPTER 16

Cheesecake

Blueberry Beauty Cheesecake

Cheesecake is one of the most loved, yet somehow most cursed fat bomb by people who don't follow a ketogenic diet. The fat content shouldn't be the blame in this situation. The high sugar content is the real crime. This version of keto cheesecake features blueberry as the star of the show.

Prep Time: 3 hours • Cook Time: 40–45 minutes

MAKES 6 FAT BOMBS

⅓ cup almond meal flour

1 tablespoon butter, melted

2 drops liquid stevia

8 ounces cream cheese, softened to room temperature

2 tablespoons granular Swerve or powdered stevia

1 large egg

½ teaspoon vanilla extract

1 tablespoon fresh lemon juice

⅓ cup fresh or frozen blueberries

Zest of ½ small lemon

1. Preheat oven to 325°F.
2. In a small mixing bowl, combine almond meal, butter, and liquid stevia.
3. Line 6 cups of a standard-sized muffin tin with cupcake liners.
4. Equally divide flour mixture between lined cups and press into bottom gently with back of a teaspoon. Prebake 10 minutes.
5. While crust is baking, thoroughly combine cream cheese and Swerve in a medium mixing bowl with a hand mixer.
6. Add egg, vanilla, and lemon juice and blend until combined.
7. Fold blueberries and lemon zest into cream cheese mixture by hand with a spatula.
8. Divide mixture between cups, return to oven, and bake another 30–35 minutes until cream cheese sets. Edges may be very slightly browned. To test doneness, insert toothpick into center of cake. If it comes out clean, cheesecake is done. Let cool and chill 2–3 hours for best flavor.

PER 1 FAT BOMB Calories: 206 | Fat: 19g | Protein: 5g | Sodium: 133mg | Fiber: 1g | Carbohydrates: 6g | Sugar: 3g

Orange Dream Cheesecake

With the addition of fresh orange, classic cheesecake takes on the flavor of a childhood favorite frozen treat, the Creamsicle. Citrus pairs well with cheese as its tartness balances the richness of the dairy.

Prep Time: 3 hours • Cook Time: 40–45 minutes

MAKES 6 FAT BOMBS

⅓ cup almond meal flour

1 tablespoon butter, melted

2 drops liquid stevia

8 ounces cream cheese, softened to room temperature

2 tablespoons granular Swerve or powdered stevia

1 large egg

½ teaspoon vanilla extract

Zest of ½ small orange

Juice of 1 small orange

1. Preheat oven to 325°F.
2. In a small mixing bowl, combine almond meal, butter, and liquid stevia.
3. Line 6 cups of a standard-sized muffin tin with cupcake liners.
4. Equally divide flour mixture between lined cups and press into bottom gently with back of a teaspoon. Prebake 10 minutes.
5. While crust is baking, thoroughly combine cream cheese and Swerve in a medium mixing bowl with a hand mixer.
6. Add remaining ingredients and blend until combined.
7. Divide mixture between cups, return to oven, and bake another 30–35 minutes until cream cheese sets. Edges may be very slightly browned. To test doneness, insert toothpick into center of cake. If it comes out clean, cheesecake is done.
8. Let cool and chill 2–3 hours for best flavor.

PER 1 FAT BOMB Calories: 211 | Fat: 19g | Protein: 5g | Sodium: 132mg | Fiber: 1g | Carbohydrates: 7g | Sugar: 4g

Lemon Lover Cheesecake

Lemon is one of the classic American flavors for drinks, pies, cakes, and treats. Adding it to a basic cheesecake elevates the dessert to a sweet and tart treat without masking the rich and creamy flavor.

Prep Time: 3 hours • Cook Time: 40–45 minutes

MAKES 6 FAT BOMBS

⅓ cup almond meal flour
1 tablespoon butter, melted
2 drops liquid stevia
8 ounces cream cheese, softened to room temperature
2 tablespoons granular Swerve or powdered stevia
1 large egg
½ teaspoon vanilla extract
Zest of ½ small lemon
Juice of 1 small lemon

1. Preheat oven to 325°F.
2. In a small mixing bowl, combine almond meal, butter, and liquid stevia.
3. Line 6 cups of a standard-sized muffin tin with cupcake liners.
4. Equally divide flour mixture between lined cups and press into bottom gently with back of a teaspoon. Prebake 10 minutes.
5. While crust is baking, thoroughly combine cream cheese and Swerve in a medium mixing bowl with a hand mixer.
6. Add remaining ingredients and blend until combined.
7. Divide mixture between cups, return to oven, and bake another 30–35 minutes until cream cheese sets. Edges may be very slightly browned. To test doneness, insert toothpick into center of cake. If it comes out clean, cheesecake is done.
8. Let cool and chill 2–3 hours for best flavor.

PER 1 FAT BOMB Calories: 203 | Fat: 19g | Protein: 5g | Sodium: 133mg | Fiber: 1g | Carbohydrates: 6g | Sugar: 2g

Divine Key Lime Cheesecake

Key lime pie is a treat beloved by many. However, keeping key limes just for pie is a bit selfish, so pairing it with cheesecake is an excellent way to spread the love. This aromatic lime elevates the cheesecake to a fresh and delicious treat.

Prep Time: 3 hours • Cook Time: 40–45 minutes

MAKES 6 FAT BOMBS

⅓ cup almond meal flour
1 tablespoon butter, melted
2 drops liquid stevia
8 ounces cream cheese, softened to room temperature
2 tablespoons granular Swerve or powdered stevia
1 large egg
½ teaspoon vanilla extract
Zest of ½ key lime
Juice of 2 key limes

1. Preheat oven to 325°F.
2. In a small mixing bowl, combine almond meal, butter, and liquid stevia.
3. Line 6 cups of a standard-sized muffin tin with cupcake liners.
4. Equally divide flour mixture between lined cups and press into bottom gently with back of a teaspoon. Prebake 10 minutes.
5. While crust is baking, thoroughly combine cream cheese and Swerve in a medium mixing bowl with a hand mixer.
6. Add remaining ingredients and blend until combined.
7. Divide mixture between cups, return to oven, and bake another 30–35 minutes until cream cheese sets. Edges may be very slightly browned. To test doneness, insert toothpick into center of cake. If it comes out clean, cheesecake is done.
8. Let cool and chill 2–3 hours for best flavor.

PER 1 FAT BOMB Calories: 207 | Fat: 19g | Protein: 5g | Sodium: 133mg | Fiber: 2g | Carbohydrates: 7g | Sugar: 2g

Vanilla Bean Cheesecake DF

For those who love cheesecake but are sensitive to dairy, this marriage of coconut and vanilla is the perfect choice. While vanilla pairs well with everything, it is an excellent companion to coconut products, lending both an aroma and flavor of the tropics.

Prep Time: 12 hours • Cook Time: 15 minutes

MAKES 6 FAT BOMBS

⅓ cup almond meal flour

1 tablespoon plus ½ cup coconut oil, melted, divided

2 drops liquid stevia

3 cups coconut milk

2 tablespoons granular Swerve or powdered stevia

½ tablespoon lemon juice

⅓ small lemon, zest only

1 teaspoon vanilla extract

1 small vanilla bean, inside scraping only

2 tablespoons powdered unflavored gelatin

⅛ teaspoon sea salt

1. Preheat oven to 350°F.
2. In a small mixing bowl, combine almond meal, 1 tablespoon coconut oil, and liquid stevia.
3. Line 6 cups of a standard-sized muffin tin with cupcake liners.
4. Equally divide flour mixture between 6 cups and press into bottom gently with back of a teaspoon. Bake 10 minutes.
5. Remove crusts from oven and let cool while making filling.
6. Combine ½ cup coconut oil, coconut milk, Swerve, lemon juice and zest, vanilla extract, and vanilla scrapings in a medium pot and heat over low heat until warmed slightly.
7. Add gelatin and salt and whisk thoroughly.
8. Remove from heat, pour into bowl, and chill in refrigerator 1 hour. Once cooled, pour into cool baked cups and return to refrigerator to chill overnight.

PER 1 FAT BOMB Calories: 455 | Fat: 47g | Protein: 6g | Sodium: 69mg | Fiber: 1g | Carbohydrates: 6g | Sugar: 5g

Pumpkin Pie Spice Cheesecake

This delicious combination of pumpkin with a cheesecake base makes the best of two American classic desserts. Opting for freshly grated nutmeg elevates the flavor of this dessert even further.

Prep Time: 3 hours • Cook Time: 40–45 minutes

MAKES 6 FAT BOMBS

⅓ cup almond meal flour

1 tablespoon butter, melted

2 drops liquid stevia

8 ounces cream cheese, softened to room temperature

2 tablespoons granular Swerve or powdered stevia

1 large egg

½ teaspoon vanilla extract

2 tablespoons puréed pumpkin

⅛ teaspoon cinnamon

⅛ teaspoon nutmeg

1. Preheat oven to 325°F.
2. In a small mixing bowl, combine almond meal, butter, and liquid stevia.
3. Line 6 cups of a standard-sized muffin tin with cupcake liners.
4. Equally divide flour mixture between lined cups and press into bottom gently with back of a teaspoon. Prebake 10 minutes.
5. While crust is baking, thoroughly combine cream cheese and Swerve in a medium mixing bowl with a hand mixer.
6. Add egg and vanilla and blend until combined.
7. Use ½ of mixture and divide equally between 6 cups.
8. Combine remaining ½ mixture with pumpkin and remaining spices until well blended. Place pumpkin mixture on top of plain layer in each cup.
9. Bake another 30–35 minutes until cream cheese sets. Edges may be very slightly browned. To test doneness, insert toothpick into center of cake. If it comes out clean, cheesecake is done.
10. Let cool and chill 2–3 hours for best flavor.

PER 1 FAT BOMB Calories: 195 | **Fat:** 18g | **Protein:** 5g | **Sodium:** 132mg | **Fiber:** 1g | **Carbohydrates:** 3g | **Sugar:** 2g

Peanut Butter Cup Cheesecake

So delicious, it's hard to believe this dessert doesn't contain sugar. The addition of natural creamy peanut butter and a chocolate drizzle gives this cheesecake the taste of a favorite peanut butter cup candy treat.

Prep Time: 3 hours • Cook Time: 40–45 minutes

MAKES 6 FAT BOMBS

⅓ cup almond meal flour

1 tablespoon butter, melted

4 drops liquid stevia, divided

8 ounces cream cheese, softened to room temperature

2 tablespoons granular Swerve or powdered stevia

1 large egg

½ teaspoon vanilla extract

2 tablespoons creamy peanut butter

1 tablespoon coconut oil, melted

1 teaspoon cocoa powder

1. Preheat oven to 325°F.
2. In a small mixing bowl, combine almond meal, butter, and 2 drops liquid stevia.
3. Line 6 cups of a standard-sized muffin tin with cupcake liners.
4. Equally divide flour mixture between lined cups and press into bottom gently with back of a teaspoon. Prebake 10 minutes.
5. While crust is baking, thoroughly combine cream cheese and Swerve in a medium mixing bowl with a hand mixer.
6. Add egg and vanilla and blend until combined.
7. Use ½ of mixture and divide equally between 6 cups.
8. Combine remaining ½ mixture with peanut butter until well blended. Take peanut butter mixture and place on top of plain layer in each cup.
9. Bake another 30–35 minutes until cream cheese sets. Edges may be very slightly browned. To test doneness, insert toothpick into center of cake. If it comes out clean, cheesecake is done.
10. Mix melted coconut oil with cocoa powder and remaining liquid stevia in a small bowl. Drizzle chocolate over top of cheesecakes.
11. Let cool and chill 2–3 hours for chocolate to set.

PER 1 FAT BOMB Calories: 245 | Fat: 24g | Protein: 6g | Sodium: 157mg | Fiber: 1g | Carbohydrates: 4g | Sugar: 2g

Taste of the Tropics Cheesecake

The use of macadamia nuts to replace a traditional gluten-based crust gives this dessert all the fat and flavor without the carbs.

Prep Time: 3 hours • Cook Time: 40–45 minutes

MAKES 6 FAT BOMBS

⅓ cup raw macadamia nuts

⅓ cup shredded unsweetened coconut

2–4 drops liquid stevia

¾ tablespoon melted butter

8 ounces cream cheese, softened to room temperature

2 tablespoons granular Swerve or powdered stevia

1 large egg

¾ teaspoon vanilla extract, divided

¼ cup canned coconut milk

¼ cup heavy whipping cream

1 teaspoon confectioners Swerve

¼ cup large-flaked toasted coconut

1. Preheat oven to 325°F. In a food processor, combine macadamia nuts, unsweetened coconut, and liquid stevia and pulse until combined. Mix in melted butter.
2. Line 6 cups of a standard-sized muffin tin with cupcake liners.
3. Equally divide nut mixture between lined cups and press into bottom gently with back of a teaspoon. Prebake 10 minutes.
4. While crust is baking, thoroughly combine cream cheese and Swerve in a medium mixing bowl with a hand mixer.
5. Add egg, ½ teaspoon vanilla, and coconut milk and blend until combined. Divide mixture equally between 6 cups.
6. Return to oven and bake another 30–35 minutes until cream cheese sets. Edges may be very slightly browned. To test doneness, insert toothpick into center of cake. If it comes out clean, cheesecake is done.
7. Let cool and chill 2–3 hours to set.
8. Just before serving, combine whipping cream, confectioners Swerve, and ¼ teaspoon vanilla in a medium bowl and beat with hand mixer until stiff peaks form. Divide equally on top of cheesecakes and sprinkle with coconut flakes.

PER 1 FAT BOMB Calories: 288 | Fat: 29g | Protein: 5g | Sodium: 139mg | Fiber: 1g | Carbohydrates: 5g | Sugar: 2g

CHAPTER 17

Sweet Mousse

Lemon Cheesecake Mousse

The delicious taste of tart lemon cheesecake meets the magical, airy texture of mousse in this fat bomb. Be sure to use fresh lemon juice and zest to give this mousse the taste of a glass of freshly squeezed lemonade.

Prep Time: 30 minutes • Cook Time: 0 minutes

SERVES 3

½ cup whipping cream

4 ounces cream cheese, softened

2 tablespoons freshly squeezed lemon juice

2 teaspoons lemon zest

1 teaspoon vanilla extract

2 tablespoons confectioners Swerve

Fresh berries, for garnish (optional)

> **A Little Bit about the Lemon**
>
> While the use of lemons can be traced back to ancient Egyptians, it became far more popular as a soft drink, known as lemonade, in the 1600s in Paris. In the mid-1800s in Italy, it starred as a frozen delight in the first known gelatos. Finally, in the late 1800s, it made it to America in lemonade stands in Brooklyn.

1. In a medium bowl, whip cream with an electric mixer until stiff peaks form.
2. In the bowl of a stand mixer, beat cream cheese, lemon juice, and lemon zest until smooth.
3. Stir in vanilla and Swerve and mix until combined. Fold in whipped cream until fully incorporated.
4. Pipe or spoon mousse into serving dishes. Refrigerate until serving. Garnish with fresh berries if desired.

PER SERVING Calories: 271 | Fat: 25g | Protein: 3g | Sodium: 135mg | Fiber: 0g | Carbohydrates: 9g | Sugar: 7g

Peanut Butter Mousse

Peanut butter is, without a doubt, one of the most purchased pantry staples, especially in homes with children. Why not use a little magic to transform this delicious fat- and protein-filled butter into a sophisticated dessert?

Prep Time: 15 minutes • Cook Time: 0 minutes

SERVES 3

½ cup heavy whipping cream, chilled
4 ounces cream cheese
2 tablespoons peanut butter
½ teaspoon vanilla extract
8 drops liquid stevia

1. Whip chilled cream in a medium bowl with a hand mixer until stiff peaks form and set aside.
2. Beat cream cheese, peanut butter, vanilla, and stevia in another medium bowl until smooth and creamy.
3. Combine whipped cream with peanut butter mixture using a hand mixer on medium speed about 1 minute or until resulting mousse is fluffy and smooth.
4. Serve immediately or store in refrigerator until ready to serve.

PER SERVING Calories: 330 | Fat: 33g | Protein: 6g |
Sodium: 184mg | Fiber: 1g | Carbohydrates: 5g | Sugar: 2g

Tiramisu Mousse

All the decadent flavor of a classic Italian dessert without the sugar-laden guilt afterward is what this mousse has to offer. Be sure to use mascarpone cheese if at all possible to get the true taste of this treasure.

Prep Time: 30 minutes • Cook Time: 0 minutes

MAKES 2 FAT BOMBS

1 teaspoon instant coffee granules

1 tablespoon hot water

½ cup heavy whipping cream

¼ cup confectioners Swerve

4 ounces mascarpone (or cream cheese if not available)

1 teaspoon vanilla extract

1 tablespoon cocoa powder

> **Pick Me Up**
> Tiramisu, the decadent Italian dessert, literally means, "pick me up." This delicious pick-me-up, unlike other Italian masterpieces, didn't make its debut until the 1970s. While it's a relative newbie to the world of desserts, its intricate flavors certainly earn this dessert its well-deserved name.

1. Dissolve coffee granules in water and let cool at least 5 minutes.
2. In a medium bowl, whip cream with an electric mixer until stiff peaks form. Set aside.
3. In another bowl, mix Swerve and mascarpone with a hand mixer until smooth.
4. Add vanilla and coffee to cheese mixture.
5. Gently fold whipped cream into cheese mixture.
6. Spoon or pipe a small amount of mousse into bottom of 2 serving glasses.
7. Top with a sprinkle of cocoa powder.
8. Repeat layers of mousse and cocoa powder until mixture is gone.
9. Cover and chill in refrigerator until ready to serve.

PER 1 FAT BOMB Calories: 312 | Fat: 28g | Protein: 3g | Sodium: 135mg | Fiber: 1g | Carbohydrates: 14g | Sugar: 11g

Peppermint Patty Mousse

Perhaps there are no two flavors that pair better together than deep dark chocolate and cooling peppermint. In this recipe, the addition of extra cocoa can make the chocolate flavor even more intense. Just be sure to add a bit more sweetener so the mousse isn't too bitter.

Prep Time: 15 minutes • Cook Time: 0 minutes

MAKES 2 FAT BOMBS
½ cup heavy whipping cream
1 teaspoon peppermint extract
¼ cup confectioners Swerve
4 ounces cream cheese, softened
1 teaspoon vanilla extract
3 tablespoons cocoa powder

1. In a small mixing bowl, mix heavy cream on high with hand blender until stiff peaks form.
2. In another bowl, mix remaining ingredients with a hand blender until smooth.
3. Fold whipped cream into cheese mixture until incorporated.
4. Place mousse into 2 serving dishes and serve immediately or cover and refrigerate until ready to serve.

PER 1 FAT BOMB Calories: 487 | Fat: 42g | Protein: 6g | Sodium: 205mg | Fiber: 3g | Carbohydrates: 24g | Sugar: 17g

Pumpkin Pie Mousse

Pumpkin pie is beloved by many, especially during the fall and winter holidays. This mousse offers a way to enjoy the unique flavor of this gourd without all the sugar, gluten, or that full gut overload of the pie.

Prep Time: 15 minutes • Cook Time: 0 minutes

MAKES 3 FAT BOMBS
½ cup heavy cream
4 ounces softened cream cheese
4 ounces canned pumpkin purée
½ teaspoon pumpkin pie spice
8 drops liquid stevia
½ teaspoon vanilla extract
½ teaspoon cinnamon (for topping)

> **Almost as American as Apple Pie**
> Although not thought of by many until Thanksgiving, pumpkin pie is actually the second most popular pie bought in stores after apple in the United States. Coming in a close third is cherry.

1. In a small mixing bowl, mix heavy cream on high with hand blender until stiff peaks form.
2. In another bowl, mix cream cheese and pumpkin with a hand blender until smooth. Add pumpkin pie spice, stevia, and vanilla and blend until combined.
3. Fold whipped cream into cheese mixture until incorporated.
4. Place mousse into 3 serving dishes and sprinkle tops with cinnamon.
5. Serve immediately or cover and refrigerate until ready to serve.

PER 1 FAT BOMB Calories: 281 | Fat: 28g | Protein: 3g | Sodium: 137mg | Fiber: 1g | Carbohydrates: 6g | Sugar: 3g

Chocolate Mousse DF

Even those who can't eat dairy can enjoy delicious chocolate mousse. Using coconut cream instead of heavy whipping cream gives this treat a subtle coconut undertone too.

Prep Time: 15 minutes • Cook Time: 0 minutes

SERVES 4

1 (13.5-ounce) can coconut milk, chilled overnight
1 tablespoon confectioners Swerve
2 tablespoons cocoa powder
⅛ teaspoon salt

1. Open can, scoop out thick cream at top, and transfer to a medium mixing bowl. (Save liquid left in bottom of can for making a smoothie later.)
2. Add Swerve and beat on high using a hand mixer about 2 minutes or until thick and creamy.
3. Reserve roughly 2 tablespoons plain whipped cream to top mousse before serving.
4. Gently fold cocoa powder and salt through whipped cream and beat again until well combined and smooth.
5. If mousse isn't set after mixing, place in refrigerate to set. Otherwise serve immediately with a dollop of plain whipped cream on top.

PER SERVING Calories: 199 | Fat: 21g | Protein: 2g | Sodium: 87mg | Fiber: 1g | Carbohydrates: 6g | Sugar: 2g

Piña Colada Mousse DF

Liking piña coladas is certainly much more appealing than "getting caught in the rain," like the old song says. This tropical-inspired mousse can be enjoyed without dairy, gluten, or added sugar.

Prep Time: 15 minutes • Cook Time: 0 minutes

MAKES 2 FAT BOMBS

1 (13.5-ounce) can coconut milk, chilled overnight

8 drops liquid stevia

½ teaspoon vanilla extract

¼ teaspoon rum extract

1 tablespoon lemon zest

⅛ teaspoon salt

2 (1") chunks freshly cut pineapple (optional)

Fun Facts about the Piña Colada

Invented in the 1950s in Puerto Rico, this tropical adult beverage actually became the national beverage of the country in 1978. The drink also has its own national holiday on July 10.

1. Open can, scoop out thick cream at top, and transfer to a medium mixing bowl. (Save liquid left in bottom of can for making a smoothie later.)
2. Add the stevia and beat on high using a hand mixer about 2 minutes or until thick and creamy.
3. Add remaining ingredients except pineapple and beat until mixture is smooth.
4. Place mousse in 2 dishes, top with pineapple, and refrigerate until set and ready to serve.

PER 1 FAT BOMB Calories: 340 | Fat: 15g | Protein: 1g | Sodium: 108mg | Fiber: 0g | Carbohydrates: 51g | Sugar: 49g

Chocolate Avocado Mousse DF

While avocado may have been popularized in America as the base for the Mexican classic guacamole, its high fat content and consistency make it an excellent choice to make a thickened dessert. Here it's combined with chocolate for a dairy-free delight.

Prep Time: 35 minutes • Cook Time: 0 minutes

MAKES 2 FAT BOMBS
½ teaspoon chia seeds (or chia powder)
2 medium avocados, pitted and peeled
8 drops liquid stevia
⅓ cup cocoa powder
2 tablespoons coconut milk

1. Grind chia seeds in a spice grinder until powdered (or use chia powder).
2. Pulse avocado in a food processor until broken down, about 1 minute.
3. Add remaining ingredients to avocado and process until smooth.
4. Scoop mixture into 2 serving dishes and refrigerate at least 30 minutes to set before serving.

PER 1 FAT BOMB Calories: 391 | Fat: 33g | Protein: 5g | Sodium: 22mg | Fiber: 20g | Carbohydrates: 33g | Sugar: 10g

CHAPTER 18

Snack Bars and Chia Puddings

Mixed-Nut Grain-Free Granola Bars DF

These treats are as tasty as granola bars without any of the grains or sugar. Another excellent addition to consider would be freeze-dried raspberries or blueberries.

Prep Time: 30 minutes • Cook Time: 20 minutes

MAKES 14 FAT BOMBS

4 ounces pumpkin seeds

4 ounces sunflower seeds

4 ounces coarsely chopped almonds

2 ounces unsweetened shredded coconut

2 ounces coconut oil, melted

4 tablespoons almond butter

1 teaspoon vanilla extract

2 teaspoons cinnamon

⅛ teaspoon salt

3 tablespoons granular Swerve

2 large eggs

> ### The Great Granola Debate
> While many health-food lovers believe granola to be an excellent nutrient-packed snack, others in the nutrition industry believe otherwise. Traditional granola, though full of fiber and iron from the granola, as well as healthy fats from the seeds and nuts, is also filled with alarming amounts of sugar, making it a less-than-healthy choice.

1. Preheat oven to 350°F.
2. Place seeds and almonds in food processor and pulse to break them up slightly.
3. Add remaining ingredients and pulse until well combined.
4. Spread mixture into an 8" × 8" silicone baking dish (or a glass dish lightly greased with coconut oil).
5. Bake 20 minutes.
6. Allow bars to cool and cut into 14 equal sections before serving.

PER 1 FAT BOMB Calories: 226 | Fat: 20g | Protein: 8g | Sodium: 54mg | Fiber: 3g | Carbohydrates: 6g | Sugar: 1g

Cinnamon Roll Bars DF

With all the flavor of a cinnamon roll and none of the gluten or sugar, this treat is sure to please even the strongest sweet tooth. Enjoy along with Po Cha (Tibetan Butter Tea; see recipe in Chapter 20) for an added treat.

Prep Time: 25 minutes • Cook Time: 0 minutes

MAKES 4 FAT BOMBS

1 cup creamed coconut, cut into chunks
1¼ teaspoons cinnamon, divided
2 tablespoons coconut oil
2 tablespoons almond butter

> **Health Benefits of Cinnamon**
> Filled with antioxidants, and anti-inflammatory in nature, cinnamon makes an excellent addition to any diet. Cinnamon is known to curb hunger, lower blood pressure, and reduce the risk of heart disease.

1. Line a mini loaf pan with parchment paper or loaf pan liners.
2. Mix creamed coconut and ¼ teaspoon cinnamon with hands thoroughly and press into bottom of loaf pan.
3. Whisk coconut oil, almond butter, and 1 teaspoon cinnamon until combined and spread over creamed coconut layer.
4. Place pan in freezer 10 minutes to set.
5. Cut into 4 equal-sized fat bombs and eat immediately.

PER 1 FAT BOMB Calories: 374 | Fat: 22g | Protein: 3g | Sodium: 64mg | Fiber: 1g | Carbohydrates: 42g | Sugar: 39g

Blueberry Coconut Cream Bars

Blueberries paired with cream cheese is no surprise to anyone who has ever had a slice of cheesecake. The addition of coconut cream gives an extra layer of fat, texture, and flavor to this delicious bar.

Prep Time: 2 hours • Cook Time: 5 minutes

MAKES 20 FAT BOMBS

1 cup fresh blueberries
8 ounces butter
¾ cup coconut oil
4 ounces cream cheese, softened
¼ cup coconut cream
¼ cup granular Swerve

1. In a small bowl, slightly crush blueberries. Pour blueberries into an 8" × 8" silicone or glass baking dish.
2. Melt butter and coconut oil over medium heat in a medium saucepan. Once melted, remove from heat and cool about 5 minutes.
3. Add remaining ingredients to saucepan and mix thoroughly with a wooden spoon.
4. Pour mixture over blueberries and place in freezer to set.
5. Remove from freezer and let warm up 15 minutes before cutting into 20 equal-sized bombs and serving.

PER 1 FAT BOMB Calories: 189 | Fat: 20g | Protein: 1g | Sodium: 21mg | Fiber: 0g | Carbohydrates: 3g | Sugar: 3g

Creamy Lemon Bars

Lemon squares are almost as delicious as lemonade. The problem with both is the incredible amount of sugar required to balance some of the tartness. The superheroes of this recipe are the Swerve and cream cheese. Now there's sweet, tart, and fat—all the ingredients for a fantastic fat bomb.

Prep Time: 30 minutes • Cook Time: 0 minutes

MAKES 8 FAT BOMBS

1 cup pecan pieces

4 ounces butter, melted

¼ cup coconut flour

3 ounces powdered unflavored gelatin

1 cup boiling water

8 ounces cream cheese, softened

2 tablespoons fresh lemon juice

1 tablespoon lemon zest

¼ cup granular Swerve

1. In a small bowl, combine pecan pieces, melted butter, and coconut flour. Spread mixture into an 8" × 8" silicone or glass baking dish and set aside.
2. Mix gelatin into boiling water in a medium bowl and stir about 2 minutes.
3. Add remaining ingredients to bowl and mix thoroughly until all lumps are gone.
4. Pour mixture over pecan crust and place in refrigerator to set. Cut into 8 bombs and serve chilled.

PER 1 FAT BOMBS Calories: 333 | Fat: 31g | Protein: 13g | Sodium: 114mg | Fiber: 4g | Carbohydrates: 6g | Sugar: 2g

Chia Energy Bars

These delicious chia bars can be a great snack before or after the gym, or for kids after school. They provide a healthy boost in energy.

Prep Time: 2 hours 15 minutes • Cook Time: 15 minutes

MAKES 14 FAT BOMBS

¼ cup chia seeds

½ cup unsweetened shredded coconut

2 tablespoons butter

¼ cup heavy cream

12 drops liquid stevia

2 tablespoons granular Swerve

1½ teaspoons vanilla extract

½ cup almond butter

½ cup coconut cream

2 tablespoons coconut flour

1 tablespoon coconut oil

1. Grind chia seeds in spice grinder until powdered. Add powder and shredded coconut to a medium pan over medium-low heat and cook until coconut is slightly brown, about 4 minutes. Set aside.

2. In a medium saucepan over medium heat, melt butter until slightly browned.

3. Turn heat to low and add heavy cream, stevia, Swerve, and vanilla and stir constantly.

4. After cream bubbles and browns, add almond butter and mix thoroughly with a wooden spoon until mixture thickens to a paste, about 5 minutes.

5. Line a 9" × 5" loaf pan with parchment paper.

6. Pour cream mixture, toasted seed mixture, coconut cream, coconut flour, and coconut oil into lined pan and mix well with fingers. Once combined, press mixture into flat sheet along bottom of pan.

7. Chill in refrigerator about 1 hour. Take out of pan, cut into 14 equal pieces, and return to refrigerator to chill another hour.

8. Serve directly from refrigerator after second chilling.

PER 1 FAT BOMB Calories: 156 | Fat: 13g | Protein: 3g | Sodium: 49mg | Fiber: 2g | Carbohydrates: 9g | Sugar: 7g

Chocolate Chia Pudding

Chocolate lover, aren't you happy you can make this fat bomb in your favorite flavor?

Prep Time: 20 minutes • Cook Time: 0 minutes

MAKES 4 FAT BOMBS

1 cup heavy cream

¼ cup chia seeds

2 tablespoons erythritol or granular Swerve

2 tablespoons cocoa powder

1 tablespoon sugar-free chocolate chips

Chia Pets or Chia Seeds?

Chia seeds not only can grow some pretty lush Chia Pets, they also have a great nutritional profile for a Keto Paleo diet. They do have about 10 percent carbohydrates, but almost all of them are pure fiber. In addition, they are a great source of omega-3 fatty acids and protein. Not bad for such little guys.

1. In a medium bowl, mix all ingredients except chocolate chips and let sit at least 15 minutes, stirring occasionally.
2. Divide among 4 cups and garnish with chocolate chips.
3. Can be stored in the refrigerator up to 3 days.

PER 1 FAT BOMB Calories: 277 | Fat: 27g | Protein: 3g | Sodium: 26mg | Fiber: 3g | Carbohydrates: 14g | Sugar: 2g

Coconut Key Lime Pie Chia Pudding

Key lime pie is a well-loved traditional recipe. This fat-bomb version will not disappoint you.

Prep Time: 20 minutes • Cook Time: 0 minutes

MAKES 4 FAT BOMBS

½ cup coconut cream

½ cup sour cream

¼ cup chia seeds

2 tablespoons erythritol or granular Swerve

1 teaspoon key lime zest

1 tablespoon fresh key lime juice

1. In a medium bowl, mix all ingredients and let sit at least 15 minutes, stirring occasionally.
2. Divide among 4 cups to serve.
3. Can be stored in the refrigerator up to 3 days.

PER 1 FAT BOMB Calories: 239 | Fat: 15g | Protein: 3g | Sodium: 40mg | Fiber: 2g | Carbohydrates: 31g | Sugar: 21g

Honey and Rose Chia Pudding DF

If you have been missing the flavor of honey, this smooth pudding, rich with creaminess and subtle aromas, will fill your senses with enjoyment.

Prep Time: 20 minutes • Cook Time: 0 minutes

MAKES 4 FAT BOMBS

1 cup coconut milk

¼ cup chia seeds

2 tablespoons erythritol or granular Swerve

4 drops honey flavor

2 tablespoons rose water

4 fresh rose petals, for garnish

1. In a medium bowl, mix all ingredients except rose petals and let sit at least 15 minutes, stirring occasionally.
2. Divide among 4 cups and garnish with rose petals.
3. Can be stored in refrigerator up to 3 days.

PER 1 FAT BOMB Calories: 157 | Fat: 16g | Protein: 3g | Sodium: 10mg | Fiber: 2g | Carbohydrates: 10g | Sugar: 0g

Raspberry and Cream Chia Pudding

Sometimes the best recipes are not difficult at all. This chia pudding is mixed together in under 3 minutes, but it will delight both children and adults.

Prep Time: 20 minutes • Cook Time: 0 minutes

MAKES 4 FAT BOMBS

1 cup heavy cream

¼ cup chia seeds

2 tablespoons erythritol or granular Swerve

4 drops raspberry flavor

2 tablespoons fresh raspberries

1. In a medium bowl, mix all ingredients except fresh raspberries and let sit at least 15 minutes, stirring occasionally.
2. Divide among 4 cups and garnish with raspberries.
3. Can be stored in refrigerator up to 3 days.

PER 1 FAT BOMB Calories: 255 | Fat: 26g | Protein: 3g | Sodium: 25mg | Fiber: 2g | Carbohydrates: 11g | Sugar: 1g

Vanilla and Cinnamon Chia Pudding

The warm spiciness of cinnamon and the sweet flavor of vanilla blend perfectly in this creamy combination.

Prep Time: 20 minutes • Cook Time: 0 minutes

MAKES 4 FAT BOMBS

1 cup heavy cream
¼ cup chia seeds
2 tablespoons erythritol or granular Swerve
1 teaspoon vanilla extract
½ teaspoon cinnamon

1. In a medium bowl, mix all ingredients and let sit at least 15 minutes, stirring occasionally.
2. Divide among 4 cups to serve.
3. Can be stored in refrigerator up to 3 days.

PER 1 FAT BOMB Calories: 257 | Fat: 26g | Protein: 3g | Sodium: 25mg | Fiber: 2g | Carbohydrates: 11g | Sugar: 0g

CHAPTER 19

Frozen Fat Bombs

Frozen Coconut White Chocolate DF

What this bomb lacks in color it more than makes up for in taste. This treat is a must make for any true lover of coconut.

Prep Time: 3 hours • Cook Time: 5 minutes

MAKES 12 FAT BOMBS

¼ cup coconut oil

¼ cup cocoa butter

1 teaspoon vanilla extract

12 drops liquid stevia

1 tablespoon unsweetened shredded coconut

1. Combine coconut oil, cocoa butter, vanilla, and stevia in a small saucepan over medium heat, stirring frequently until ingredients have melted. Turn off heat.
2. Add coconut and stir well to combine.
3. Pour mixture into 12 molds of a silicone-bottomed ice cube tray or silicone candy mold tray until about ¾ full.
4. Freeze until set. Serve from freezer.

PER 1 FAT BOMB Calories: 82 | Fat: 9g | Protein: 0g | Sodium: 0mg | Fiber: 0g | Carbohydrates: 0g | Sugar: 0g

Frozen Almond Choco-Nut DF

Although this fat bomb tastes like a familiar candy bar, this knockoff is full of fat and flavor and very low in carbs. This bomb would also be delicious without the added almonds.

Prep Time: 3 hours • Cook Time: 5 minutes

MAKES 12 FAT BOMBS

¼ cup coconut oil

¼ cup almond butter

12 drops liquid stevia

2 tablespoons cocoa powder

¼ cup coarsely chopped almonds

1 tablespoon unsweetened shredded coconut

> **Mounds Sports a Two-Piece**
>
> Although not common knowledge to younger generations, Mounds candy bars were originally sold as one piece, not two. Sometime in the 1970s, the creator Peter Paul broke the bar into two pieces, lowered the weight of the candy by an ounce, and raised the price by a nickel.

1. Combine coconut oil, almond butter, and stevia in a small pot over medium heat, stirring frequently until ingredients have melted. Turn off heat.
2. Add cocoa powder and almonds and stir well to combine.
3. Pour mixture into 12 molds of a silicone-bottomed ice cube tray or silicone candy mold tray until about ¾ full.
4. Sprinkle shredded coconut on top of each fat bomb.
5. Freeze until set. Serve from freezer.

PER 1 FAT BOMB Calories: 87 | Fat: 8g | Protein: 2g | Sodium: 25mg | Fiber: 1g | Carbohydrates: 2g | Sugar: 1g

Frozen Maca-Nutty Bites DF

What better way to make macadamia nuts even more tasty than to drench them in chocolate? These tasty bites work best when poured into silicone candy trays or silicone-bottomed ice cube trays.

Prep Time: 3 hours • Cook Time: 5 minutes

MAKES 12 FAT BOMBS

¼ cup coconut oil
¼ cup almond butter
1 teaspoon vanilla extract
12 drops liquid stevia
2 tablespoons cocoa powder
12 whole macadamia nuts

1. Combine coconut oil, almond butter, vanilla, and stevia in a small saucepan over medium heat, stirring frequently until ingredients have melted. Turn off heat.
2. Add cocoa powder and stir well to combine.
3. Pour mixture into 12 molds of a silicone-bottomed ice cube tray or silicone candy mold tray until about ⅔ full.
4. Place 1 macadamia nut into each filled mold.
5. Freeze until set. Serve from freezer.

PER 1 FAT BOMB Calories: 93 | Fat: 9g | Protein: 2g |
Sodium: 25mg | Fiber: 1g | Carbohydrates: 2g | Sugar: 1g

Frozen Coffee Hazelnut Coconut DF

Here's another way to enjoy the bold taste of coffee on the go as a delicious cold treat. This bomb is an easy way to replace those expensive sugar-filled iced coffees that are so readily available.

Prep Time: 3 hours • Cook Time: 5 minutes

MAKES 12 FAT BOMBS

¼ cup coconut oil
¼ cup almond butter
1 teaspoon instant coffee granules
12 drops liquid stevia
2 tablespoons cocoa powder
12 hazelnuts

1. Combine coconut oil, almond butter, coffee, and stevia in a small saucepan over medium heat, stirring frequently until ingredients have melted. Turn off heat.
2. Add cocoa powder and stir well to combine.
3. Pour mixture into 12 molds of a silicone-bottomed ice cube tray or silicone candy mold tray until about ⅔ full.
4. Place 1 hazelnut into each filled mold.
5. Freeze until set. Serve from freezer.

PER 1 FAT BOMB Calories: 96 | Fat: 8g | Protein: 2g | Sodium: 25mg | Fiber: 1g | Carbohydrates: 2g | Sugar: 1g

Frozen Butter Rum Chocolate DF

For those who love the taste of rum but not the added calories of alcohol, this is a handy treat. While it is possible to use actual rum for this dessert, the use of an extract is highly recommended to reduce the intake of unwanted sugar.

Prep Time: 3 hours • Cook Time: 5 minutes

MAKES 12 FAT BOMBS

¼ cup coconut oil

¼ cup almond butter

2 teaspoons rum extract

12 drops liquid stevia

2 tablespoons cocoa powder

1. Combine all ingredients except cocoa powder in a small saucepan over medium heat, stirring frequently until ingredients have melted. Turn off heat.
2. Add cocoa powder and stir well to combine.
3. Pour mixture into 12 molds of a silicone-bottomed ice cube tray or silicone candy mold tray until about ¾ full.
4. Freeze until set. Serve from freezer.

PER 1 FAT BOMB Calories: 75 | Fat: 7g | Protein: 2g | Sodium: 25mg | Fiber: 1g | Carbohydrates: 2g | Sugar: 1g

The American Colonists' Drink of Choice Was Rum and Chocolate

Early American colonists drank rum as their primary alcoholic beverage, which is no surprise due to the Caribbean rum trade. But would you picture those same colonists drinking chocolate? It's true. Long before eating chocolate became popular, American colonists drank it.

Frozen Salted Caramel Almond

Golden, creamy, delicious caramel is nothing more than butter, sugar, and cream. This dairy- and sugar-free version sets up quite well in the freezer, making it an excellent substitute for its sugar-filled twin.

Prep Time: 3 hours • Cook Time: 5 minutes

MAKES 12 FAT BOMBS

¼ cup butter
¼ cup granular Swerve
2 teaspoons vanilla extract
12 whole almonds
1 teaspoon coarse sea salt

1. Combine butter, Swerve, and vanilla in a small saucepan over medium heat, stirring frequently until ingredients have melted. Turn off heat.
2. Place 1 almond into each mold of a 12-mold silicone candy tray.
3. Carefully pour mixture over each of the almonds until molds are about ¾ full.
4. Sprinkle salt on top of each fat bomb.
5. Freeze until set. Serve from freezer.

PER 1 FAT BOMB Calories: 64 | Fat: 7g | Protein: 0g | Sodium: 296mg | Fiber: 0g | Carbohydrates: 1g | Sugar: 0g

Frozen Orange Creamsicle

The sounds of a good old-fashioned ice cream truck jingle fill the air with just the thought of making this fat bomb. Cream cheese plays a much needed role to add body and support to this treat.

Prep Time: 3 hours • Cook Time: 0 minutes

MAKES 12 FAT BOMBS

¼ cup coconut oil

¼ cup heavy whipping cream

2 ounces cream cheese, softened

2 tablespoons freshly squeezed orange juice

1 tablespoon orange zest

12 drops liquid stevia

> **National Creamsicle Day Does Exist**
>
> Although not recognized as an official holiday on the American calendar, this treat is so popular that August 14 is known as National Creamsicle Day. The Creamsicle was further developed from the 1905 creation of the Popsicle by Frank Epperson.

1. Combine all ingredients in a small wide-mouthed jar or bowl and blend with an immersion blender, about 30 seconds.
2. Spread mixture into 12 molds of a silicone candy mold tray.
3. Freeze until set. Serve from freezer.

PER 1 FAT BOMB Calories: 75 | Fat: 8g | Protein: 0g | Sodium: 17mg | Fiber: 0g | Carbohydrates: 1g | Sugar: 0g

Frozen Matcha Cream DF

These wonderful treats will give your energy a big boost, both through the ketone-producing MCT (medium-chain triglyceride) oils in the coconut and through the caffeine in the matcha.

Prep Time: 3–12 hours • Cook Time: 5 minutes

MAKES 12 FAT BOMBS

Ganache

3 ounces cocoa butter

3 ounces coconut cream

1 tablespoon coconut oil

½ teaspoon matcha

2 tablespoons confectioners Swerve

2 drops stevia glycerite

⅛ teaspoon sea salt

Coating

2 tablespoons matcha

1. In a small double boiler (bain-marie) over medium-low heat, melt cocoa butter while stirring slowly.
2. Add coconut cream, coconut oil, ½ teaspoon matcha, Swerve, stevia, and sea salt and mix well until incorporated.
3. Remove from heat and keep stirring about 10 seconds.
4. Pour into a silicone mold for chocolate or candy in the desired shape. Molds should be about 1" deep and 1½" wide.
5. Freeze at least 3 hours or overnight. Once frozen, remove shapes from molds then sprinkle with 2 tablespoons matcha to coat tops. Can be stored in a sealed container in freezer or refrigerator.

PER 1 FAT BOMB Calories: 103 | Fat: 9g | Protein: 0g | Sodium: 291mg | Fiber: 0g | Carbohydrates: 6g | Sugar: 5g

Frozen Coconut Rum DF

A flavor fit for a vacation under palm trees. Let yourself be transported to an island with the first bite.

Prep Time: 3–12 hours • Cook Time: 5 minutes

MAKES 10 FAT BOMBS

Ganache

2 ounces cocoa butter

2 ounces coconut cream

2 tablespoons confectioners Swerve

¼ teaspoon rum flavor

2 drops stevia glycerite

4 tablespoons unsweetened shredded coconut

Coating

2 tablespoons shredded coconut

Silicone Molds

You can use fun silicone molds to make your frozen treats into shapes like hearts or sea shells. Just pour the ganache straight from the saucepan into the molds and then freeze until solid. When ready, remove from the mold and roll in coating agent. They're ready to eat!

1. In a small double boiler (bain-marie) over medium-low heat, melt cocoa butter while stirring slowly.
2. Add coconut cream, Swerve, rum flavor, stevia, and 4 tablespoons shredded coconut and mix well until incorporated.
3. Remove from heat and keep stirring about 10 seconds.
4. Pour into a silicone mold for chocolate or candy in desired shape. Molds should be about 1" deep and 1½" wide.
5. Freeze at least 3 hours or overnight. Once frozen, remove ganache shapes from molds then sprinkle with 2 tablespoons shredded coconut to coat tops. Can be stored in a sealed container in freezer or refrigerator.

PER 1 FAT BOMB Calories: 86 | Fat: 8g | Protein: 0g | Sodium: 3mg | Fiber: 0g | Carbohydrates: 5g | Sugar: 5g

Almond Cookie Popsicles DF

*Sweet and creamy almond flavor, no sugar, and lots of healthy fat.
And no dairy, so if you are dairy sensitive you can enjoy this too!*

Prep Time: 8–12 hours • Cook Time: 0 minutes

MAKES 8 FAT BOMBS

1½ cups coconut cream, chilled
½ cup almond butter
1 teaspoon vanilla extract
¼ cup erythritol or granular Swerve

1. Place all ingredients in a blender and blend until completely mixed, about 30 seconds.
2. Pour mix into 8 popsicle molds, tapping molds to dislodge air bubbles.
3. Freeze at least 8 hours or overnight.
4. Remove popsicles from molds. If popsicles are hard to remove from containers, run molds under hot water briefly and popsicles will come loose.

PER 1 FAT BOMB Calories: 294 | Fat: 17g | Protein: 5g | Sodium: 94mg | Fiber: 1g | Carbohydrates: 39g | Sugar: 30g

Butter Pecan Popsicles

An old-time favorite flavor, these Butter Pecan Popsicles are a great way to cool off after a long summer day . . . especially when you need more fat and have had enough carbs for the day.

Prep Time: 8–12 hours • Cook Time: 5 minutes

MAKES 8 FAT BOMBS

2 tablespoons butter

1 cup coarsely chopped pecans

3 tablespoons erythritol or granular Swerve, divided

1½ cups heavy cream

1 teaspoon vanilla extract

⅛ teaspoon salt

1. In a medium nonstick pan over medium heat, melt butter. Then add pecans and 1 tablespoon sweetener and cook about 3 minutes. Set aside to cool.
2. In a blender, mix cream, 2 tablespoons sweetener, vanilla, and salt about 10 seconds.
3. Scoop cooled pecans into bottom of 8 popsicle molds, dividing them equally.
4. Pour cream mix into molds, tapping molds to dislodge air bubbles.
5. Freeze at least 8 hours or overnight.
6. Remove popsicles from molds. If popsicles are hard to remove from containers, run molds under hot water briefly and popsicles will come loose.

PER 1 FAT BOMB Calories: 276 | Fat: 29g | Protein: 2g | Sodium: 54mg | Fiber: 1g | Carbohydrates: 8g | Sugar: 1g

Chocolate-Drizzled Creamy Peanut Butter Popsicles

Peanut butter and chocolate . . . a very kid-friendly combination. Your kids will enjoy this popsicle as much as you do, and they're a great alternative to traditional sugary snacks as well.

Prep Time: 8–12 hours • Cook Time: 8 minutes

MAKES 8 FAT BOMBS

½ cup mascarpone
½ cup unsweetened peanut butter
1 cup heavy cream
2 tablespoons erythritol or granular Swerve
1 teaspoon vanilla extract
2 ounces unsweetened baking chocolate
1 tablespoon confectioners Swerve

1. In a small saucepan over low heat, combine mascarpone, peanut butter, and cream. Stir until melted, about 3 minutes. Set aside to cool.

2. In a blender, add cream mixture, sweetener, and vanilla. Blend until combined, about 10 seconds.

3. Pour cream mix into molds, tapping molds to dislodge air bubbles.

4. Freeze at least 8 hours or overnight.

5. In a double boiler over medium-low heat, melt chocolate and confectioners Swerve.

6. Remove popsicles from molds. If popsicles are hard to remove from containers, run molds under hot water briefly and popsicles will come loose.

7. With a spoon, drizzle melted chocolate over each popsicle and serve immediately.

PER 1 FAT BOMB Calories: 288 | Fat: 28g | Protein: 6g | Sodium: 134mg | Fiber: 2g | Carbohydrates: 11g | Sugar: 3g

Coconut Vanilla Popsicles DF

A simple, clean flavor to please even the most picky eaters. Kids will love this popsicle.

Prep Time: 8–12 hours • Cook Time: 0 minutes

MAKES 8 FAT BOMBS

2 cups coconut cream, chilled
¼ cup unsweetened shredded coconut
1 teaspoon vanilla extract
¼ cup erythritol or granular Swerve

1. Place all ingredients in a blender and blend until completely mixed, about 30 seconds.
2. Pour mix into 8 popsicle molds, tapping molds to dislodge air bubbles.
3. Freeze at least 8 hours or overnight.
4. Remove popsicles from molds. If popsicles are hard to remove from containers, run molds under hot water briefly and popsicles will come loose.

PER 1 FAT BOMB Calories: 274 | Fat: 13g | Protein: 1g |
Sodium: 27mg | Fiber: 0g | Carbohydrates: 46g | Sugar: 38g

Dark Chocolate Popsicles DF

You will be amazed at the smooth, rich, chocolaty flavor of this popsicle. Nobody will ever suspect there is an avocado in there.

Prep Time: 8–12 hours • Cook Time: 0 minutes

MAKES 4 FAT BOMBS

1 medium avocado, pitted and peeled
½ cup coconut cream
⅓ cup cocoa powder
3 tablespoons erythritol or granular Swerve
⅛ teaspoon vanilla extract
⅛ teaspoon salt

1. Place all ingredients in a small food processor or blender and blend until completely mixed, about 30 seconds.
2. Pour mix into 4 popsicle molds, tapping molds to dislodge air bubbles.
3. Freeze at least 8 hours or overnight.
4. Remove popsicles from molds. If popsicles are hard to remove from containers, run molds under hot water briefly and popsicles will come loose.

PER 1 FAT BOMB Calories: 229 | Fat: 14g | Protein: 3g | Sodium: 92mg | Fiber: 6g | Carbohydrates: 37g | Sugar: 20g

Ginger Cream Popsicles DF

A very similar flavor to the chewy ginger candy, without the sugar and with a good dose of healthy fat!

Prep Time: 8–12 hours • Cook Time: 0 minutes

MAKES 8 FAT BOMBS

2 cups coconut cream, chilled

2 tablespoons coconut oil

1 teaspoon ground ginger

¼ cup erythritol or granular Swerve

Ginger Power

Ginger is not only a delicious flavor for both sweet and savory dishes, but it is also a medicinal root. It has great digestive proprieties, it prevents gas, and it is most effective at eliminating nausea.

1. Place all ingredients in a blender and blend until completely mixed, about 30 seconds.
2. Pour mix into 8 popsicle molds, tapping molds to dislodge air bubbles.
3. Freeze at least 8 hours or overnight.
4. Remove popsicles from molds. If popsicles are hard to remove from containers, run molds under hot water briefly and popsicles will come loose.

PER 1 FAT BOMB Calories: 295 | Fat: 15g | Protein: 1g | Sodium: 27mg | Fiber: 0g | Carbohydrates: 46g | Sugar: 38g

Hazelnut Cappuccino Popsicles

Do you love a steamy, fragrant cappuccino with hazelnut syrup? In the heat of summer, you will love this popsicle version.

Prep Time: 8–12 hours • Cook Time: 1 minute

MAKES 8 FAT BOMBS

1 cup brewed espresso or strong coffee
1 cup heavy whipping cream
⅛ teaspoon hazelnut flavor
¼ cup erythritol or granular Swerve
½ cup crumbled hazelnuts

1. Place all ingredients except hazelnuts in a blender and blend until completely mixed, about 30 seconds.
2. Pour mix into 8 popsicle molds, tapping molds to dislodge air bubbles.
3. Freeze at least 8 hours or overnight.
4. In a small nonstick pan over medium heat, toast crumbled hazelnuts about 1 minute, stirring constantly.
5. Remove popsicles from molds. If popsicles are hard to remove from containers, run molds under hot water briefly and popsicles will come loose.
6. Before serving, press popsicles into hazelnut crumbles so they coat the outside.

PER 1 FAT BOMB Calories: 148 | Fat: 15g | Protein: 2g | Sodium: 11mg | Fiber: 1g | Carbohydrates: 8g | Sugar: 0g

Matcha Popsicles DF

Creamy, refreshing, and with the energizing qualities of matcha, this is a delicious popsicle for grownups.

Prep Time: 8–12 hours • Cook Time: 0 minutes

MAKES 8 FAT BOMBS

2 cups coconut cream, chilled
2 tablespoons coconut oil
1 teaspoon matcha
¼ cup erythritol or granular Swerve

1. Place all ingredients in a blender and blend until completely mixed, about 30 seconds.
2. Pour mix into 8 popsicle molds, tapping molds to dislodge air bubbles.
3. Freeze at least 8 hours or overnight.
4. Remove popsicles from molds. If popsicles are hard to remove from containers, run molds under hot water briefly and popsicles will come loose.

PER 1 FAT BOMB Calories: 294 | Fat: 15g | Protein: 1g | Sodium: 88mg | Fiber: 0g | Carbohydrates: 46g | Sugar: 38g

Green Rocket Fuel

Matcha is a finely ground powder of a specially grown green tea. Matcha is basically a form of whole green tea leaves with extra theanine and chlorophyll. It also contain high levels of catechin antioxidants, and a good amount of caffeine. As matcha contains the whole leaf, you also get fiber and a higher content of nutrients than regular brewed green tea.

Mint Chocolate Chip Popsicles

Whether you call it mint chip or chocolate mint, this flavor has a lot of loyal fans. In fact, it is quoted as one of the ten most popular ice cream flavors. This popsicle version should make the fans even happier.

Prep Time: 8–12 hours • Cook Time: 5 minutes

MAKES 8 FAT BOMBS

2 cups coconut cream
1 cup fresh mint leaves
2 ounces unsweetened chocolate chips
¼ cup erythritol or granular Swerve

1. Combine coconut milk and mint in a medium saucepan over medium heat.
2. Simmer until bubbles start appearing, about 5 minutes. Remove from heat and let steep 20 minutes.
3. Strain through a fine-mesh sieve into a bowl.
4. Add chocolate and sweetener and stir well.
5. Pour mix into 8 popsicle molds, tapping molds to dislodge air bubbles.
6. Freeze at least 8 hours or overnight.
7. Remove popsicles from molds. If popsicles are hard to remove from containers, run molds under hot water briefly and popsicles will come loose.

PER 1 FAT BOMB Calories: 304 | Fat: 16g | Protein: 2g | Sodium: 32mg | Fiber: 2g | Carbohydrates: 48g | Sugar: 38g

Orange Chocolate Popsicles DF

This tangy treat is a sensation to savor. The rich chocolate flavor blended with a delicate hint of citrus will leave everyone smiling.

Prep Time: 8–12 hours • Cook Time: 0 minutes

MAKES 4 FAT BOMBS

1 medium avocado, pitted and peeled
½ cup coconut cream
½ cup cocoa powder
2 tablespoons erythritol or granular Swerve
1 teaspoon orange zest
⅛ teaspoon orange extract
⅛ teaspoon salt

1. Place all ingredients in a small food processor or blender and blend until completely mixed, about 30 seconds.
2. Pour mix into 4 popsicle molds, tapping molds to dislodge air bubbles.
3. Freeze at least 8 hours or overnight.
4. Remove popsicles from molds. If popsicles are hard to remove from containers, run molds under hot water briefly and popsicles will come loose.

PER 1 FAT BOMB Calories: 237 | Fat: 15g | Protein: 4g | Sodium: 93mg | Fiber: 7g | Carbohydrates: 36g | Sugar: 20g

CHAPTER 20

Drinks and Smoothies

Amaretto Chilled Coffee

What a delightful treat for a summer evening. Instead of a cocktail, enjoy this cool and satisfying fat bomb.

Prep Time: 8 minutes • Cook Time: 0 minutes

MAKES 2 FAT BOMBS

2 cups cooled brewed coffee

4 teaspoons erythritol or granular Swerve, or 3 drops stevia glycerite, divided

4 drops amaretto flavor, divided

½ cup heavy cream, chilled

1 teaspoon crumbled roasted almonds

1. Pour coffee into a medium bowl and mix with half the sweetener and half the amaretto flavor.
2. In a blender add chilled cream, remaining amaretto flavor, and remaining sweetener. Blend on high until cream is whipped.
3. When ready to serve, pour coffee mix over ice in 2 glasses.
4. Spoon whipped cream on top of coffee mix. Decorate with chopped almonds.
5. Serve immediately with a spoon and a straw.

PER 1 FAT BOMB Calories: 421 | Fat: 23g | Protein: 12g | Sodium: 55mg | Fiber: 0g | Carbohydrates: 45g | Sugar: 0g

Coconut Coffee

This coffee recipe is a great way to introduce healthy fat early in your day.

Prep Time: 1 minute • Cook Time: 0 minutes

MAKES 1 FAT BOMB

1½ cups hot brewed coffee

2 teaspoons erythritol or granular Swerve, or 2 drops stevia glycerite

1 tablespoon coconut oil

1 tablespoon butter

⅛ teaspoon sea salt

1. Place all ingredients in a blender.
2. Blend on high about 15 seconds.
3. Serve immediately.

PER 1 FAT BOMB Calories: 534 | Fat: 28g | Protein: 16g | Sodium: 344mg | Fiber: 0g | Carbohydrates: 61g | Sugar: 0g

Caffeine-Free Coconut Vanilla Tea DF

A hot drink that is a breakfast in itself, this recipe does not have caffeine or dairy, so it is suitable for the strictest of diets.

Prep Time: 2 minutes • Cook Time: 8 minutes

MAKES 1 FAT BOMB

1 teabag rooibos tea

1½ cups hot water

2 teaspoons erythritol or granular Swerve, or 2 drops stevia glycerite

1 tablespoon coconut oil

⅛ teaspoon vanilla extract (optional)

1. Place teabag in water and brew about 8 minutes.
2. Place brewed tea in a blender with remaining ingredients.
3. Blend on high 15 seconds.
4. Serve immediately.

PER 1 FAT BOMB Calories: 135 | Fat: 14g | Protein: 0g | Sodium: 11mg | Fiber: 0g | Carbohydrates: 8g | Sugar: 0g

Creamy Mexican Hot Chocolate

Mexican chocolate is a true indulgence: rich and thick with a touch of cinnamon flavor. You can serve this sugar-free version to your family and they will love it any time of year. Try it this fall next to a blazing campfire.

Prep Time: 3 minutes • Cook Time: 5 minutes

MAKES 2 FAT BOMBS

1 cup water

1 cup heavy cream

2 teaspoons erythritol or granular Swerve, or 2 drops stevia glycerite

⅓ cup cocoa powder

1 teaspoon cinnamon

⅛ teaspoon vanilla extract

4 tablespoons unsweetened whipped cream

1. In a small saucepan over very low heat, combine all ingredients except whipped cream.
2. Heat while stirring constantly until cocoa powder is completely dissolved, about 5 minutes. Do not boil.
3. When ready to serve, pour chocolate into 2 cups and top with whipped cream.

PER 1 FAT BOMB Calories: 538 | Fat: 56g | Protein: 6g | Sodium: 63mg | Fiber: 5g | Carbohydrates: 17g | Sugar: 0g

Po Cha (Tibetan Butter Tea)

Tibetan butter tea is originally made with yak butter and a potent brew of smoky tea leaves. You do not have to look for yak butter to recreate this flavorful drink at home; you'll still reap all the benefits of starting your day off right with a high-fat treat.

Prep Time: 3 minutes • Cook Time: 8 minutes

MAKES 2 FAT BOMBS

4 cups water
2 tablespoons black tea leaves
2 tablespoons butter
2 tablespoons heavy cream
⅛ teaspoon sea salt
1 drop smoke flavor

> **The Original Recipe**
> This is the recipe that originally inspired the Bulletproof concept. This Tibetan recipe is a staple of their culture. Butter tea, known as *po cha* in Tibetan, is consumed every day, multiple times a day. The drink has many benefits, including giving warmth to the drinker and providing a stable, longlasting energy source, which is much needed at high altitudes.

1. In a small saucepan over high heat, bring water to a boil, then lower heat to low.
2. Add tea leaves to water and simmer about 3 minutes. Strain.
3. Combine brewed tea with remaining ingredients in a blender and mix on high about 3 minutes.
4. Serve immediately.

PER 1 FAT BOMB Calories: 153 | Fat: 17g | Protein: 0g | Sodium: 169mg | Fiber: 0g | Carbohydrates: 0g | Sugar: 0g

Thai Iced Coffee

Every Thai restaurant serves some version of this drink. Now you can enjoy this version, which is full of beneficial fat.

Prep Time: 5 minutes • Cook Time: 0 minutes

MAKES 2 FAT BOMBS

4 cups strong brewed coffee, cooled

4 teaspoons erythritol or granular Swerve, or 3 drops stevia glycerite

2 tablespoons coconut milk

⅛ teaspoon vanilla extract

4 tablespoons heavy cream

1. Pour coffee into a large bowl and mix with sweetener, coconut milk, and vanilla.
2. Pour coffee mixture over ice in 2 tall glasses. Pour cream on top of coffee without stirring so layers remain separate.
3. Serve immediately with a tall spoon and a straw.

PER 1 FAT BOMB Calories: 548 | Fat: 15g | Protein: 22g | Sodium: 77mg | Fiber: 0g | Carbohydrates: 80g | Sugar: 0g

Creamy Coconut Smoothie DF

Feel free to add a splash of rum extract and a pineapple wedge.

Prep Time: 5 minutes • Cook Time: 0 minutes

MAKES 1 FAT BOMB

½ (13.5-ounce) can coconut milk

1 tablespoon powdered unflavored gelatin

1 tablespoon coconut oil, softened but not melted

1 teaspoon vanilla extract

1 tablespoon unsweetened shredded coconut

6 drops liquid stevia

6 ice cubes

1. Pour milk and gelatin into a blender and blend to combine.
2. Add remaining ingredients except ice cubes and blend another minute until well mixed.
3. Place ice cubes into blender and process until smoothie thickens. Serve immediately.

PER 1 FAT BOMB Calories: 559 | Fat: 57g | Protein: 10g | Sodium: 41mg | Fiber: 0g | Carbohydrates: 7g | Sugar: 1g

Thai Iced Tea

A great variation of Thai iced coffee. It's great during the heat of summer, but should be enjoyed year-round.

Prep Time: 15 minutes • Cook Time: 8 minutes

MAKES 2 FAT BOMBS

4 cups water

2 tablespoons Ceylon variety black tea leaves

2 cardamom pods, crushed

1 teaspoon star anise seeds

2 teaspoons erythritol or granular Swerve, or 2 drops stevia glycerite

4 tablespoons heavy cream

2 tablespoons coconut milk

⅛ teaspoon vanilla extract

1. In a small saucepan over high heat, bring water to a boil, then lower heat to low.
2. Add tea leaves, cardamom, and anise seeds and simmer about 3 minutes. Strain.
3. Let brewed tea cool, then pour over ice in 2 tall glasses.
4. In a small bowl combine sweetener, cream, coconut milk, and vanilla and stir well until sweetener has dissolved.
5. Pour cream mix on top of tea without stirring so layers remain separate.
6. Serve immediately with a tall spoon and a straw.

PER 1 FAT BOMB Calories: 144 | Fat: 15g | Protein: 1g | Sodium: 28mg | Fiber: 1g | Carbohydrates: 7g | Sugar: 0g

Blueberry Chocolate Smoothie DF

Blueberries covered in dark chocolate, while delicious, are full of sugar. The darker the chocolate, the sweeter blueberries taste. While this smoothie has no sugar, it certainly is not short on taste.

Prep Time: 5 minutes • Cook Time: 0 minutes

MAKES 1 FAT BOMB

½ (13.5-ounce) can coconut milk

1 tablespoon powdered unflavored gelatin

1 tablespoon coconut oil, softened but not melted

2 tablespoons cocoa powder

¼ cup frozen blueberries

6 drops liquid stevia

6 ice cubes

A Natural Food Dye

Blueberries are not only a tasty lower-carbohydrate fruit, but they make an excellent natural food dye. You can just blend them into a recipe to add blue color! A blueberry, when first picked, however, should be dusty in color.

1. Pour milk and gelatin into a blender and blend to combine.
2. Add remaining ingredients except ice cubes and blend another minute until well mixed.
3. Place ice cubes into blender and process until smoothie thickens. Serve immediately.

PER 1 FAT BOMB Calories: 560 | Fat: 55g | Protein: 12g | Sodium: 41mg | Fiber: 5g | Carbohydrates: 16g | Sugar: 3g

Cinnamon Roll Smoothie

The only difference between the sugar- and gluten-filled version of the roll and this smoothie is the time it takes to make it, and of course the fact that it fits into a low-carb, high-fat diet.

Prep Time: 5 minutes • Cook Time: 0 minutes

MAKES 1 FAT BOMB

6 ounces half-and-half

1 tablespoon softened cream cheese

1 teaspoon vanilla extract

½ teaspoon plus ⅛ teaspoon cinnamon, divided

6 drops liquid stevia

6 ice cubes

> **More Popular Than IKEA**
> While it may be an enormously popular American breakfast staple, the cinnamon roll was actually created in Sweden. Next to these delicious fried cinnamon treats, furniture would be Sweden's second most popular export.

1. Pour half-and-half and cream cheese into a blender and blend to combine.
2. Add vanilla, ½ teaspoon cinnamon, and stevia and blend another minute until well mixed.
3. Place ice cubes into blender and process until smoothie thickens. Sprinkle ⅛ teaspoon cinnamon on top and serve.

PER 1 FAT BOMB Calories: 283 | Fat: 24g | Protein: 6g | Sodium: 116mg | Fiber: 1g | Carbohydrates: 9g | Sugar: 1g

Eggnog Smoothie

Traditional eggnog would make an excellent choice for a fat bomb, if it wasn't for all the sugar included. This smoothie has all the fat and flavor without the added carbs.

Prep Time: 10 minutes • Cook Time: 0 minutes

MAKES 2 FAT BOMBS

2 large eggs, yolk and white separated
8 ounces heavy cream
½ teaspoon vanilla extract
1 teaspoon nutmeg
⅛ teaspoon ground cloves
⅜ teaspoon cinnamon, divided
8 drops liquid stevia
2 tablespoons granular Swerve
8 ice cubes

1. In a medium bowl, beat egg whites with a hand mixer until stiff peaks form. Set aside.
2. In a separate large bowl, beat yolks with mixer until color changes to pale yellow. Add cream, vanilla, nutmeg, cloves, ⅛ teaspoon cinnamon, stevia, and Swerve and stir to combine.
3. Fold whites into yolk mixture.
4. Pour mix into blender with ice cubes and blend until mixture thickens.
5. Sprinkle ⅛ teaspoon cinnamon on top of each glass and serve immediately.

PER 1 FAT BOMB Calories: 468 | Fat: 47g | Protein: 9g | Sodium: 113mg | Fiber: 1g | Carbohydrates: 5g | Sugar: 1g

Gingerbread Gem Smoothie DF

Ginger is an often forgotten spice in American cuisine unless it's Christmastime. This delicious, dairy-free smoothie will taste and smell like a Christmas cookie bake-off.

Prep Time: 5 minutes • Cook Time: 0 minutes

MAKES 1 FAT BOMB

6 ounces unsweetened almond milk

1 tablespoon powdered unflavored gelatin

1 tablespoon almond butter

½ teaspoon vanilla extract

½ teaspoon ground ginger

½ teaspoon cinnamon

6 drops liquid stevia

6 ice cubes

1. Pour milk and gelatin into a blender and blend to combine.
2. Add remaining ingredients except ice cubes and blend another minute until well mixed.
3. Place ice cubes into blender and process until smoothie thickens. Serve immediately.

PER 1 FAT BOMB Calories: 221 | Fat: 11g | Protein: 16g | Sodium: 174mg | Fiber: 3g | Carbohydrates: 16g | Sugar: 9g

Key Lime Pie Smoothie

Using full-fat dairy lends richness to this tropical-tasting treat.

Prep Time: 5 minutes • Cook Time: 0 minutes

MAKES 1 FAT BOMB

6 ounces half-and-half

1 tablespoon powdered unflavored gelatin

1 teaspoon vanilla extract

2 tablespoons freshly squeezed key lime (or regular lime) juice

1 teaspoon lime zest

6 drops liquid stevia

6 ice cubes

1. Pour half-and-half and gelatin into a blender and blend to combine. Add remaining ingredients except ice cubes and blend another minute until well mixed.
2. Place ice cubes into blender and process until smoothie thickens. Serve immediately.

PER 1 FAT BOMB Calories: 280 | Fat: 20g | Protein: 12g | Sodium: 91mg | Fiber: 2g | Carbohydrates: 17g | Sugar: 3g

Peanut Butter Cup Smoothie DF

Love the candy treat but not the sugar? This smoothie is truly the drinkable version, ready in minutes for breakfast on the go.

Prep Time: 5 minutes • Cook Time: 0 minutes

MAKES 1 FAT BOMB

½ (13.5-ounce) can coconut milk

1 tablespoon powdered unflavored gelatin

2 tablespoons peanut butter

2 tablespoons cocoa powder

1 teaspoon vanilla extract

6 drops liquid stevia

4 ice cubes

1. Pour milk and gelatin into a blender and blend to combine.
2. Add remaining ingredients except ice cubes and blend another minute until well mixed.
3. Place ice cubes into blender and process until smoothie thickens. Serve immediately.

PER 1 FAT BOMB Calories: 622 | Fat: 58g | Protein: 20g | Sodium: 189mg | Fiber: 6g | Carbohydrates: 18g | Sugar: 4g

Matcha Madness Smoothie DF

Matcha not only adds antioxidants to this smoothie, but also a beautiful green hue. The best quality matcha powders add a bit of earthy flavor and a subtle sweetness too.

Prep Time: 5 minutes • Cook Time: 0 minutes

MAKES 1 FAT BOMB
½ (13.5-ounce) can coconut milk
1 tablespoon powdered unflavored gelatin
2 tablespoons almond butter
1 teaspoon vanilla extract
1 tablespoon matcha
6 drops liquid stevia
4 ice cubes

1. Pour milk and gelatin into a blender and blend to combine.
2. Add remaining ingredients except ice cubes and blend another minute until well mixed.
3. Place ice cubes into blender and process until smoothie thickens. Serve immediately.

PER 1 FAT BOMB Calories: 610 | Fat: 57g | Protein: 19g | Sodium: 187mg | Fiber: 4g | Carbohydrates: 15g | Sugar: 4g

Orange Delight Smoothie

This shake has the taste of a Creamsicle without the unnecessary sugar.

Prep Time: 5 minutes • Cook Time: 0 minutes

MAKES 1 FAT BOMB

6 ounces half-and-half

1 tablespoon powdered
  unflavored gelatin

1 teaspoon vanilla extract

2 tablespoons freshly squeezed
  orange juice

1 teaspoon orange zest

4 drops liquid stevia

6 ice cubes

1. Pour half-and-half and gelatin into a blender and blend to combine. Add remaining ingredients except ice cubes and blend another minute until well mixed.
2. Place ice cubes into blender and process until smoothie thickens. Serve immediately.

PER 1 FAT BOMB Calories: 271 | Fat: 19g | Protein: 11g | Sodium: 84mg | Fiber: 0g | Carbohydrates: 12g | Sugar: 4g

Strawberry Vanilla Smoothie DF

Strawberries are a great fruit to up the flavor of any smoothie without adding too much sugar.

Prep Time: 5 minutes • Cook Time: 0 minutes

MAKES 1 FAT BOMB

½ (13.5-ounce) can coconut milk

1 tablespoon powdered
  unflavored gelatin

1 tablespoon coconut oil,
  softened but not melted

1 teaspoon vanilla extract

¼ cup chopped fresh strawberries

6 drops liquid stevia

6 ice cubes

1. Pour milk and gelatin into a blender and blend to combine. Add remaining ingredients except ice cubes and blend another minute until well mixed.
2. Place ice cubes into blender and process until smoothie thickens. Serve immediately.

PER 1 FAT BOMB Calories: 540 | Fat: 54g | Protein: 10g | Sodium: 39mg | Fiber: 1g | Carbohydrates: 9g | Sugar: 2g

Vanilla Avocado Smoothie DF

Avocado not only adds body to this smoothie, it makes this smoothie a beautiful green color too. Of course, the healthy omega-3 fats make this shake an even more filling fat bomb.

Prep Time: 5 minutes • Cook Time: 0 minutes

MAKES 1 FAT BOMB

½ (13.5-ounce) can coconut milk
1 tablespoon powdered unflavored gelatin
1 tablespoon ground flaxseed
½ medium avocado, pitted and peeled
1 teaspoon vanilla extract
6 drops liquid stevia
4 ice cubes

1. Pour milk, gelatin, and flaxseed into a blender and blend to combine.
2. Add remaining ingredients except ice cubes and blend another minute until well mixed.
3. Place ice cubes into blender and process until smoothie thickens. Serve immediately.

PER 1 FAT BOMB Calories: 603 | Fat: 57g | Protein: 14g | Sodium: 46mg | Fiber: 9g | Carbohydrates: 17g | Sugar: 1g

Vanilla Almond Butter Smoothie DF

Almond butter is a fantastic way to boost fat, protein, and thickness in a smoothie. The addition of a few drops of almond extract can actually boost the nutty flavor if preferred over vanilla.

Prep Time: 5 minutes • Cook Time: 0 minutes

MAKES 1 FAT BOMB

6 ounces unsweetened almond milk

1 tablespoon powdered unflavored gelatin

2 tablespoons almond butter

1 teaspoon vanilla extract

¼ teaspoon almond extract (optional)

6 drops liquid stevia

4 ice cubes

1. Pour milk and gelatin into a blender and blend to combine.
2. Add remaining ingredients except ice cubes and blend another minute until well mixed.
3. Place ice cubes into blender and process until smoothie thickens. Serve immediately.

PER 1 FAT BOMB Calories: 316 | Fat: 19g | Protein: 19g | Sodium: 248mg | Fiber: 3g | Carbohydrates: 17g | Sugar: 10g

Avocado Almond Smoothie DF

The avocado in this recipe will make your smoothie nice and creamy without masking the almond flavor.

Prep Time: 3 minutes • Cook Time: 0 minutes

MAKES 2 FAT BOMBS

1 cup coconut milk

½ large avocado, pitted and peeled

¼ cup ice

1 teaspoon almond extract

4 drops liquid stevia

2 tablespoons coconut butter

Combine all ingredients in blender and blend until smooth. Serve immediately.

PER 1 FAT BOMB Calories: 423 | Fat: 45g | Protein: 3g | Sodium: 18mg | Fiber: 3g | Carbohydrates: 7g | Sugar: 0g

Very Vanilla Smoothie

The best way to elevate the "plain vanilla" milkshake is to use fresh vanilla bean in place of extract. Using vanilla bean makes this smoothie a tastier choice than even the best ice cream shop masterpiece.

Prep Time: 5 minutes • Cook Time: 0 minutes

MAKES 1 FAT BOMB

6 ounces half-and-half

1 tablespoon powdered unflavored gelatin

1 teaspoon vanilla extract

1 vanilla bean, scraped, pulp only

4 drops liquid stevia

6 ice cubes

> **Unusual Uses for Vanilla**
>
> Vanilla is a delicious flavor to add to many treats, but it is far more versatile than that. Vanilla can be used to freshen the smell in a refrigerator, cool a burn, and even to repel insects.

1. Pour half-and-half and gelatin into a blender and blend to combine.
2. Add remaining ingredients except ice cubes and blend another minute until well mixed.
3. Place ice cubes into blender and process until smoothie thickens. Serve immediately.

PER 1 FAT BOMB Calories: 274 | Fat: 19g | Protein: 11g | Sodium: 83mg | Fiber: 0g | Carbohydrates: 8g | Sugar: 1g

Special Instructions for Fat-Bomb Cooking

Dividing Coconut Milk for Coconut Cream

The easiest way to get coconut cream is to get a (13.5-ounce) can of full-fat organic coconut milk and put it in the refrigerator overnight. In the morning, flip the can upside down and open it. Pour out the coconut water, which contains most of the sugar, then scoop out the cream, which will be now solid. You can use this cream in any recipe that calls for coconut cream.

Cooking Prosciutto and Making Prosciutto Crumbles

To get prosciutto crumbles, pre-heat oven to 350°F. Place thin prosciutto slices on a cookie sheet and bake about 12 minutes. Remove from oven and let cool. Once cold and crispy, chop finely with a sharp kitchen knife until reduced to crumbles.

Cooking Bacon

There are two simple ways you can prepare your bacon for any of the recipes in this book:

Pan-Frying Method

Place the bacon slices closely together in a cold frying pan. Cook over medium heat without moving the slices about 5 minutes. The bacon should by then move easily and not be stuck to the bottom of the pan. Flip the bacon and cook about 5 more minutes. Remove from the pan and drain on a paper towel.

Oven Method

Preheat oven to 400°F. Place a rack inside a baking sheet. Lay the bacon slices on the rack and bake 10–15 minutes, depending on desired doneness level.

Ketogenic Shopping List

Fats and Oils

- Avocado oil
- Avocados
- Butter
- Coconut butter
- Coconut flakes (unsweetened)
- Coconut milk (full-fat)
- Coconut oil
- Olive oil
- Olives

Protein

- Bacon
- Canned salmon
- Canned tuna
- Deli meat: prosciutto, pepperoni, turkey, roast beef, ham (make sure there is no added sugar)
- Eggs
- Fresh fish: cod, salmon, halibut, mackerel, herring, sardines, tuna, anchovies (wild-caught is best)
- Meat: beef, veal, venison, bison, lamb (grass-fed is best)
- Pork: pork loin, ham, pork chops (humanely treated, pastured is best; make sure ham contains no sugar)
- Poultry: chicken, turkey, duck (free-range is best)
- Sausage
- Shellfish: shrimp, crab, lobster, scallops, mussels, oysters, clams

Dairy Products

- Asiago cheese
- Cheddar cheese
- Cottage cheese
- Cream cheese
- Heavy cream
- Mozzarella cheese
- Parmesan cheese
- Pepper jack cheese
- Ricotta cheese
- Sour cream

Fruits

- Blackberries
- Blueberries
- Granny Smith apples
- Lemons
- Raspberries

Vegetables

- Asparagus
- Baby kale
- Bell peppers
- Broccoli
- Brussels sprouts
- Cabbage
- Cauliflower
- Celery
- Cucumbers
- Eggplant
- Garlic
- Lettuce (iceberg and romaine)
- Mushrooms
- Onions
- Scallions
- Shallots
- Spaghetti squash
- Spinach
- Tomatoes (canned whole and fire-roasted diced)
- Zucchini

Nuts, Nut Butters, and Seeds

- Almond butter
- Almonds
- Cashew butter
- Cashews
- Chia seeds
- Macadamia nuts
- Peanut butter
- Peanuts
- Pecans
- Pistachio nuts
- Pumpkin seeds
- Sunflower seeds
- Walnuts

Condiments

- Apple cider vinegar
- Hot sauce
- Mustard
- Pickles
- White vinegar

Sweeteners and Extracts

- Almond extract
- Erythritol (granulated and powdered)
- Orange extract
- Peppermint extract
- Stevia (liquid and granulated)
- Vanilla extract

Miscellaneous

- Cocoa powder (unsweetened)
- Dark chocolate
- Pork rinds
- Whey protein powder (sugar-free—low net carbohydrates)

Resources

The Nourished Caveman

http://thenourishedcaveman.com

The Nourished Caveman is a food blog and valuable resource for all things keto. Find recipes, health guidance, FAQs, and keto products, and more.

Boston Children's Hospital

300 Longwood Avenue
Fegan 9
Boston, MA 02115
(617) 355-6815
www.childrenshospital.org

Boston Children's Hospital has a Pediatric Epilepsy Program that can provide support for children with epilepsy. Their program is rated as a Level 4 Epilepsy Center by the National Association of Epilepsy Centers because they deliver an extremely high level of care that includes the use of the ketogenic diet.

Children's Hospital Los Angeles

4650 Sunset Blvd.
Los Angeles, CA 90027
(323) 361-8531
www.chla.org

Children's Hospital Los Angeles specializes in pediatrics and uses the classic ketogenic diet and modified ketogenic diet as part of their epilepsy treatment program.

Keto Calculator

http://keto-calculator.ankerl.com

Easily calculate your macronutrient ratios for the ketogenic diet with this online diet calculator.

The Charlie Foundation

515 Ocean Avenue
#602N
Santa Monica, CA 90402
(310) 393-2347
www.charliefoundation.org

The Charlie Foundation provides information and dietary therapies for people with epilepsy, other neurological disorders, and cancer.

The Institute for Functional Medicine

505 S. 336th Street
Suite 600
Federal Way, WA 98003
(800) 228-0622
www.functionalmedicine.org

The goal of the Institute for Functional Medicine is to reverse chronic disease and advance knowledge by providing information and education about functional medicine.

The UltraWellness Center

Dr. Mark Hyman
55 Pittsfield Road
Suite 9
Lenox Commons, Lenox, MA 01240
(413) 637-9991
www.ultrawellnesscenter.com

Dr. Mark Hyman is one of the leaders in functional medicine. He founded the UltraWellness Center in Lenox, Massachusetts, and has authored several books.

INDEX